T0280848

This concise yet immensely practical handbook provides the busy clinician with a self-contained account of the diagnosis and management of ectopic pregnancy. Such pregnancies, which develop outside the normal confines of the uterine cavity, are a relatively common occurrence and there is some evidence their incidence is increasing. There is therefore a need for a practical and focused account which assesses and evaluates the important clinical issues. The emphasis throughout is to clearly summarise and provide rapid solutions to the most difficult problems posed by ectopic pregnancy. The text is fully supported by numerous and helpful ultrasound images, line diagrams illustrating surgical techniques, and by highlighted summaries of key facts and decision trees.

Ectopic pregnancy

Ectopic pregnancy: diagnosis and management

ISABEL STABILE

Professor, Center for Biomedical Research, Florida State University

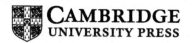

CAMBRIDGE
UNIVERSITY PRESS

Published by the Press Syndicate of the University of Cambridge
The Pitt Building, Trumpington Street, Cambridge CB2 1RP
40 West 20th Street, New York, NY 10011-4211, USA
10 Stamford Road, Oakleigh, Melbourne 3166, Australia

© Cambridge University Press 1996

First published 1996

A catalogue record for this book is available from the British Library

Library of Congress cataloguing in publication data

Stabile, Isabel, 1957–
   Ectopic pregnancy : diagnosis and management / Isabel Stabile.
     p. cm.
  ISBN 0 521 49612 8 (pbk.)
    1. Ectopic pregnancy. I. Title.
    [DNLM: 1. Pregnancy, Ectopic – diagnosis. 2. Pregnancy,
Ectopic – therapy. WQ 220 S775e 1996]
  RG586.S83 1996
  618.3'1 – dc20
  DNLM/DLC
  for Library of Congress 95–21096 CIP

ISBN 0 521 49612 8 paperback

Transferred to digital printing 2003

CONTENTS

CHAPTER 1

Incidence, aetiology and pathophysiology of ectopic pregnancy

1.1   Definition

Tubal, ectopic and extrauterine are terms used to describe pregnancies occurring outside the uterine cavity. While tubal pregnancies are located strictly within the fallopian tube, the latter two terms include ovarian and abdominal pregnancies, as well as those implanting in the oviduct. An ovum may be fertilised and remain at any point along its passage from the ovary to the uterus (Figure 1.1).

1.2   Incidence: is it increasing?

The incidence of ectopic pregnancy ranges between 0.25% and 1.4% of all pregnancies, i.e. the sum of reported live births, legal induced abortions and ectopic pregnancies (Chow *et al.*, 1987; Coste *et al.*, 1994). Controversy has arisen over the ideal denominator in reporting the incidence of ectopic pregnancy (Box 1.1). Barnes and colleagues (1983) have shown that the estimated rate of ectopic pregnancy in New England can vary up to 35-fold depending on the denominator used. Another limitation in accurately identifying ectopic pregnancy rates is the problem of ensuring that the diagnosis is not missed, especially in very early cases which may spontaneously resolve. Comparative rates of ectopic pregnancy in France, Finland and the USA are listed in Table 1.1. In 1992, ectopic pregnancies accounted for approximately 2% of reported pregnancies in the USA and ectopic pregnancy-related deaths accounted for 9% of all pregnancy-related deaths (NCHS, 1994). The estimated total number of ectopic pregnancies obtained from inpatient and outpatient data was 47% higher than that obtained from hospitalisations only (MMWR, 1995).

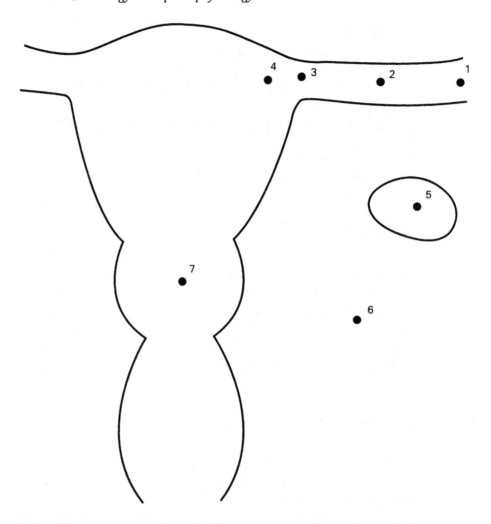

Figure 1.1 Possible implantation sites in ectopic pregnancy. 1, ampulla; 2, isthmus; 3, interstitial portion; 4, angular portion; 5, ovary; 6, peritoneum; 7, cervix.

Whatever the incidence of ectopic pregnancy and however it is defined, there is no doubt that it is increasing worldwide. In Finland for example the annual number of cases more than tripled from 1966 to 1985 (Makinen *et al.*, 1989), while in the USA, the Centers for Disease Control have reported a fourfold increase in the incidence of ectopic pregnancy between 1970 and 1989 (CDC, 1986, 1992). This has led some to speak of an epidemic, although the term is not strictly accurate as 'epidemic' should be used to describe short outbreaks of large numbers of cases. Ectopic pregnancy has always been endemic (widespread in large numbers over a long period of time in the community). In many ways the

---

Box 1.1. Choice of denominator in defining the incidence of ectopic pregnancy (EP).

1. Live births
   - Advantages: easy to collect; usually accurate
   - Disadvantages: birth rates vary; excludes women who choose abortion if they become pregnant; patients with EP are not strictly a subset of this denominator
2. 10 000 women aged 14–44 years
   - Advantages: well defined in census data; low risk population at extremes of age; eliminates those not at risk of pregnancy complications; meaningful where abortion is illegal or not reported; includes that subset of women having EP
   - Disadvantages: increasing risk of infertility with advancing age; more widespread use of contraception
3. Total no. of conceptions including all abortions, spontaneous and induced
   - Advantages: includes that subset of women having EP
   - Disadvantages: difficult to obtain accurately because spontaneous abortions are often under-reported
4. Reported pregnancies
   - Advantages: easy to collect; includes subset of women having EP

Table 1.1. *Comparative rates of ectopic pregnancy in France, Finland and the USA*

	Reference	Per 1000 live births	Per 1000 reported pregnancies	Per 10000 women aged 15–44 years
France	Coste *et al.* (1994)	20.2	15.8	9.5
Finland	Makinen (1993)	28	21	16.3
USA	CDC (1992)	22	16.1	15.5

epidemiology is similar to that of infectious diseases: there are epidemics, well-established long-term trends and known distributions within geographical and socio-economic categories. For example, a higher incidence is recorded in Jamaica (one in 28 deliveries) and in Saigon (one in 40 deliveries), probably reflecting the lower socio-economic status and the higher incidence of pelvic inflammatory disease (PID) in these communities (Stabile and Grudzinskas, 1990). For reasons unknown, ectopic pregnancy is reportedly less frequent in spring and summer than in autumn and winter (Coste *et al.*, 1994).

1.3   Who is at risk?

All sexually active women are at risk of ectopic pregnancy, but in some a combination of factors puts them at much higher risk. In this respect it is important to distinguish between association and causation. The factors listed in Box 1.2 increase the risk of ectopic pregnancy, but it is not always clear what role they play in the aetiology of the condition (Chow *et al.*, 1987). For example, 4–8% of all accidental pregnancies with the unmedicated intrauterine contraceptive device (IUD) *in situ* are ectopic gestations (Vessey *et al.*, 1974; Tatum and Schmidt, 1977). The likelihood of ectopic pregnancy increases as the duration of IUD use increases (Ory, 1981), perhaps because the IUD causes deciliation, especially after 3 years or more of use (Wollen *et al.*, 1984). This may explain why the predisposition to ectopic pregnancy remains after the IUD is removed (Vessey *et al.*, 1974). Although the postulated association of IUDs with ectopic pregnancy is theoretically attractive (and is possibly modulated by intervening PID which causes physical changes in the fallopian tube), it is not universally accepted that the IUD is the prime cause (Sivin, 1983). Indeed, there is mounting evidence that the IUD *in situ* reduces the absolute likelihood of ectopic pregnancy. For example, the multicentre case control study of Ory (1981) showed that current IUD users had the same risk as never-users of IUDs for ectopic pregnancy and that if the IUD were used for more than 25 months the user was 2.6 times more likely to have an ectopic pregnancy than a short-term user. In the case controlled study of the World Health Organization (WHO) (1985), current IUD users were six times more likely to experience an ectopic pregnancy than pregnant controls (who are less likely to have an IUD in place) but only half as likely to have an ectopic pregnancy as non-pregnant controls.

Lehfeldt and colleagues (1970) have shown that the IUD reduces the risk of intrauterine pregnancy by 99.5%, the risk of tubal pregnancy by 95% and that of ovarian pregnancy not at all, thus accounting for the relative increase in tubal and ovarian pregnancy in IUD users. The incorporation of a progestogen into the inert device appears to increase further the incidence of ectopic pregnancy (Snowden, 1977). Rossing *et al.* (1993) have demonstrated that current contraceptive users (including IUD and oral contraceptives) are much less likely (relative risk of 0.2 for IUD users) to experience an ectopic pregnancy than are non-users of contraceptives.

In conclusion, in spite of numerous studies, the relationship between IUD use and ectopic pregnancy remains controversial. This is in part

---

Box 1.2. Who is at risk?

The cause of ectopic pregnancy remains an enigma but several risk factors and associated conditions have been implicated. The highest incidence is in:

- Women with a history of a previous ectopic pregnancy
- Documented previous salpingitis resulting in tubal damage
- Women with a history of infertility
- Previous pelvic surgery including sterilisation
- Women aged 35 years or older
- Races other than white
- IUD users
- Exposure to diethylstilboestrol *in utero*

---

because the risk of IUD use differs for current users compared with past users and because information about past use is difficult to interpret, for example, some past IUD users are currently using other methods of contraception which may alter risk.

1.4 Why does ectopic pregnancy occur? Distinguishing fact from fiction

The aetiology of ectopic pregnancy remains an enigma. The major cause is destruction of the anatomy of the tube which leads to altered tubal transport. Other causes are listed in Box 1.3 and include unusual length of the tubes, kinking and diverticula. It is suggested that as the ovum now has to make a longer journey than usual, it may have become too large to pass through the tube, or the development of the trophoblast may be so far advanced that implantation of the fertilised ovum begins. One of the oldest theories is that salpingitis is the major cause of ectopic pregnancy: the loss of the ciliated epithelium and induration of the tubal musculature impeding propulsion of the ovum. Adhesions between neighbouring folds of mucous membrane are thought to form cul-de-sacs, from which the ovum cannot escape. The chief argument against salpingitis as a major cause is that in many cases there is no evidence of inflammation in the walls of the fallopian tubes. The evidence for and against PID as a cause of ectopic pregnancy is summarised in Box 1.4. The question of why ectopic pregnancy also occurs in histologically normal tubes is considered in Box 1.5.

Box 1.3. Controversial causes of ectopic pregnancy.

1. Psychological stress causing tubal spasm
2. Congenital abnormalities
3. Blind tubal pouches (diverticula)
4. Leiomyomata
5. Endometriosis
6. Poor semen quality
7. Abnormal prostaglandin levels in semen
8. Smoking
9. Vaginal douching

Box 1.4. Does pelvic inflammatory disease (PID) cause ectopic pregnancy (EP)?

Evidence for:
- Westrom *et al* 1981: Case-controlled study reporting a sevenfold increase in EP rate following laparoscopically verified acute salpingitis
- Current increase in EP incidence parallels increase in salpingitis
- Documented mechanism available: acute/chronic inflammation results in obstruction to passage of fertilised ovum
- Histologically normal tubes removed for EP have marked decrease in ciliated cells on EM, an abnormality seen also in patients with documented PID
- Patients with EP have higher *Chlamydia trachomatis* specific IgG titre than controls

Evidence against:
- Only 50% of tubal specimens removed for EP have evidence of chronic salpingitis by H&E staining

---

Studies on the causes of ectopic pregnancy are hampered by the lack of a good experimental model because the condition is rare even in higher primates. Much work has been carried out in rodents but these lower mammals are highly resistant to tubal implantation, perhaps because metabolic activation of the embryo (a prerequisite for trophoblast invasion) is impaired within the non-human oviduct.

1.5   How do intrauterine and extrauterine implantation differ?

The ratio of ectopic pregnancy to intrauterine pregnancy is estimated to be between 1:84 and 1:230 (Elias *et al.*, 1981). Although less likely than

---

Box 1.5. Why does ectopic pregnancy (EP) occur in histologically normal tubes?

Possible mechanisms include:
1. Under-reporting of inflammation
2. Altered transport mechanisms:
   - (a) Progestogens decrease ciliation and slow down ovum transport
   - (b) High oestrogens may immobilise cilia and alter smooth muscle contractility
3. Altered embryo quality:
   - (a) Chromosomal abnormalities
   - (b) Higher frequency of anembryonic pregnancies in EP
4. Delayed ovulation and/or short or inadequate luteal phase
5. Transperitoneal migration of fertilised ovum

---

intrauterine pregnancy in any woman, the fact that ectopic pregnancy is more common with advancing age raises the possibility that abnormal embryogenesis might be more common in ectopic gestation than in spontaneous abortion. Bearing in mind the limitations of any morphological or karyotypic study of ectopic gestations (embryo absent or macerated, failure of cultures to grow, biased reporting of one particular type of abnormality or failure to control for confounders such as smoking, drinking and parity), the limited evidence suggests that the percentage of abnormal embryos in ectopic pregnancy (approximately one-third) is no different from that in spontaneous intrauterine abortions of the same gestational age (Poland and Kalousek, 1986). Moreover, approximately 50% of ectopic pregnancies are anembryonic (Emmrich and Kopping, 1981), a figure which is similar to that documented by detailed ultrasonic study of spontaneous intrauterine abortions (Stabile *et al.*, 1989). Thus if an embryo is present within a tubal gestational sac, it is no more likely to be abnormal than an embryo implanting within the uterus.

Differences between implantation in the uterus and in the tube can be explained by anatomical differences between these two organs. In healthy tubes only a very thin layer of connective tissue separates the epithelium from the muscle, whereas the uterine endometrium forms a thick vascular layer into which the ovum can sink. The trophoblast invades the muscle of the tube but there is no decidua formation comparable to that which occurs in the uterus to limit the destructive action of the trophoblast. As growth continues, the connective tissue cells of the tube wall may become swollen and resemble decidual cells; however, these provide no resistance to the invading trophoblast. If the trophoblast encounters and invades larger blood vessels, the pressure of the blood stream is often sufficient to destroy the embryonic cell mass.

The early development of the tubal placenta is very similar to that seen in the uterus, although it is often immature and many villi demonstrate the loss of vascularity and central hyalinisation which is characteristic of collapse of the fetal circulation. Subsequently there is failure of the tubal trophoblast to differentiate into a chorion laevae and chorion frondosum. Decidual reaction around the tubal implantation site is usually minimal. At the appropriate stage of development, the human blastocyst can implant at a variety of sites, primarily as a result of trophoblastic activity; maternal tissues play only a passive role.

1.6   Morphology of the ectopic conceptus

Embryonic death and tubal abortion are the most common outcome of tubal pregnancies. A live embryo is found in up to 20% of ectopic pregnancies, even when transvaginal sonography (TVS) is used. In the remaining cases, there is either partial or complete absence of the embryo (50%) or one or more morphological abnormalities. There are no significant differences in either morphological or chromosomal features among ectopic and failed intrauterine pregnancies of the same gestational age (Elias *et al.*, 1981; Poland and Kalousek, 1986).

Once the trophoblast implants on the tubal mucosa it may invade the lamina propria and tubal musculature to grow in the potential space between the wall of the oviduct and the peritoneum; under these circumstances the wall is very likely to rupture (Figure 1.2). Alternatively its growth may be predominantly intraluminal. The latter is most likely with implantation in the ampulla and the former with implantation in the isthmus (Senterman *et al.*, 1988). A mixed pattern may also occur. As the pregnancy continues there is penetration of tubal blood vessels, choriodecidual haemorrhage and early separation of the products of conception from the implantation site (Section 1.5). This leads to embryonic death, cessation of trophoblastic activity and tubal abortion.

Tubal abortion occurs in one of three ways.

1. There may be spontaneous regression of the pregnancy with resorption of the products of conception and the surrounding haematoma. Innovations in ultrasound technology have revealed that this so-called missed tubal abortion (or tubal mole) is probably more common than was once thought. Management of these cases should be conservative.

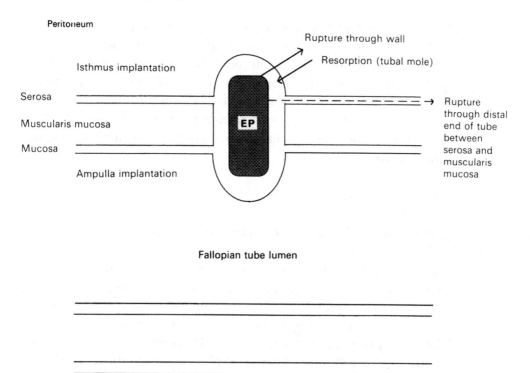

Peritoneum

Rupture through wall

Isthmus implantation

Resorption (tubal mole)

Serosa

Rupture through distal end of tube between serosa and muscularis mucosa

Muscularis mucosa

EP

Mucosa

Ampulla implantation

Fallopian tube lumen

Figure 1.2 Diagrammatic section through fallopian tube showing possible implantation sites of ectopic conceptus and outcomes.

2. There may be circumferential growth of the conceptus with bleeding and expulsion of the products of conception through the distal end of the tube between the fimbrial tissue and the serosa (rather than through the lumen of the tube) into the peritoneal cavity. As in uterine abortion, this process may be complete or incomplete, the latter being accompanied by continued bleeding from the end of the tube. Gradual accumulation of blood may form a pelvic haematocoele presenting with recurrent abdominal pain and vaginal bleeding. After a complete tubal abortion the tube resumes its normal appearance. Probably many cases of this type pass unnoticed. Fimbrial evacuation or milking of tubal pregnancies, although easy to perform, is often followed by repeat ectopic pregnancy; the process may cause increased tubal destruction because of preferential growth of the conceptus within the oviduct wall. Some would reserve the term tubal abortion for this process of internal rupture of the gestational sac, just as rupture of the tube is an external rupture.

3. Tubal rupture may occur when the serosa is stretched to its limit. Rupture may be sudden, the patient becoming profoundly collapsed in

a few minutes, or more commonly it may be gradual as the tubal wall is slowly eroded by the trophoblast. Rupture and the accompanying haemorrhage may occur into the peritoneal cavity (intraperitoneal rupture), or occasionally between the layers of the broad ligament (extraperitoneal rupture). Intraperitoneal rupture of an isthmic ectopic may occur even before a menstrual period is missed. Tubal rupture is now uncommon because of earlier diagnosis and recourse to surgical management.

1.7   A special case: heterotopic pregnancy

Heterotopic pregnancy is the combined occurrence of intrauterine and extrauterine gestations. The incidence in spontaneous conceptions was originally estimated at one in 30000 gestations (De Voe and Pratt, 1948), but more recent evidence suggests that the incidence lies between 1:4000 to 1:7000 of all pregnancies (Hahn *et al.*, 1984; Reece *et al.*, 1983). It is significantly higher following *in vitro* fertilisation and embryo transfer (IVF-ET), the reported rate ranging from 1% to 3% of all clinical pregnancies and 10–15% of all IVF-ET ectopic gestations (Rizk *et al.*, 1991). This rate is most likely related to transferring a larger number of embryos (Tummon *et al.*, 1994). In women undergoing abortion, the death to case rate from concurrent ectopic pregnancy is reportedly 1.3 times higher than that for women not undergoing abortion (Atrash *et al.*, 1990).

Since the first report of the ultrasonographic demonstration of heterotopic pregnancy (Penkava and Behling, 1979), the diagnosis is being made earlier by recourse to TVS. The diagnosis is often delayed because the symptoms are attributed to the complications of intrauterine pregnancy. The levels of human chorionic gonadotrophin (hCG) are often in the normal range. Abortion of the intrauterine pregnancy may precede or follow rupture of the ectopic gestational sac. Early diagnosis, therefore, is on the basis of maintaining a high index of suspicion, particularly following gamete manipulation, pelvic surgery or a history of pelvic inflammatory disease, although cases have been reported in women without any risk factors (Jerrard *et al.*, 1992).

Heterotopic pregnancy remains a difficult diagnostic and management problem, and will not be diagnosed unless it is considered in all patients with the classical symptomatology of ectopic pregnancy, even when an intrauterine pregnancy has been visualised ultrasonically. Although the diagnosis is being made earlier by TVS (Mattox *et al.*, 1989), laparoscopy is often helpful. This should be followed by the least invasive therapeutic regimen available to ensure continuing viability of the intrauterine pregnancy.

1.8   Point summary

1. Approximately 1% of all pregnancies are ectopic.

2. There has been a worldwide increase in incidence in the past 25 years.

3. The risk of ectopic pregnancy is increased in association with previous pelvic surgery, salpingitis and a previous ectopic pregnancy as well as in women undergoing assisted conception.

4. The incidence of abnormal embryos is similar in ectopic pregnancy and spontaneous abortion.

5. Implantation and early placentation are similar in ectopic and intrauterine pregnancy.

6. Embryonic death and tubal abortion are the most common outcomes of tubal pregnancy.

7. Heterotopic pregnancy is commoner than once thought (approximately 1:4000 pregnancies).

1.9   References

Atrash H.K., MacKay, H.T., Hogue, C.J. (1990). Ectopic pregnancy concurrent with induced abortion: incidence and mortality. *American Journal of Obstetrics and Gynecology* **162**(3): 726–730.

Barnes, A.B., Wennberg, C.N., Barnes, B.A. (1983). Ectopic pregnancy: incidence and review of determinant factors. *Obstetrics and Gynecology Survey*, **38**: 345–356.

CDC (Centers for Disease Control) (1986). Ectopic pregnancy in the USA: 1970–1983, CDC surveillance summaries. *Morbidity and Mortality Weekly Report*, **35**: 29.

CDC (Centers for Disease Control) (1992). Ectopic pregnancy in the USA, 1978–1989, CDC surveillance summaries. *Morbidity and Mortality Weekly Report*, **41**: 591–594.

Chow, W.H., Daling, J.R., Cates, W., Greenberg, R.S (1987). Epidemiology of ectopic pregnancy. *Epidemiology Review*, **9**: 70–94.

Coste, J., Job-Spira, N., Aublet-Cuvelier, B., Germain, E., Glowaczower, E., Fernandez, H., Pouly, J.L. (1994). Incidence of ectopic pregnancy. First results of a population-based register in France. *Human Reproduction*, **9**: 742–745.

De Voe, R., Pratt, J. (1948). Simultaneous intra- and extrauterine pregnancy. *American Journal of Obstetrics and Gynecology*, **56**: 1119–1125.

Elias, S., LeBeau, M., Simpson, J.L., Martin, A.O. (1981). Chromosomal analysis of ectopic human conceptuses. *American Journal Obstetrics and Gynecology*, **141**: 698–703.

Emmrich, P., Kopping, H. (1981). A study of placental villi in extrauterine gestation: a guide to the frequency of blighted ova. *Placenta*, **2**: 63–70.

Hahn, L., Bachman, D., McArdle, C. (1984). Co-existent intrauterine and ectopic pregnancy. A re-evaluation. *Radiology*, **152**: 151–154.

Jerrard, D., Tso, E., Salik, R., Barish, R.A. (1992). Unsuspected heterotopic pregnancy in a woman without risk factors. *American Journal of Emergency Medicine*, **10**(1), 58–60.

Lehfeldt, H., Tietze, C., Gorstein, F. (1970). Ovarian pregnancy and the intrauterine device. *American Journal Obstetrics and Gynecology*, **108**: 1005–1009.

Makinen, J. (1993). Is the epidemic of ectopic pregnancy over? In *Proceedings of the 10th Meeting of the International Society for STD Research*, Helsinki, Finland, 29 August–1 September, 1993, pp. 71–79

Makinen, J., Erkkola, R.U., Laippala, P.J. (1989). Causes of the increase in incidence of ectopic pregnancy: a study on 1017 patients from 1966 to 1985 in Turku, Finland. *American Journal Obstetrics and Gynecology*, **160**: 642–646.

Mattox, J.H., Kolb, D.J., Goggin, M.W., Thomas, W.E. (1989). Heterotopic pregnancy diagnosed by endovaginal scanning. *Journal of Clinical Ultrasound*, **17**(7): 523–526.

Morbidity and Mortality Weekly Report. (1995). Current trend in ectopic pregnancy, US 1990–1992. *Morbidity and Mortality Weekly Report*, CDC, 95/01/29.

NCHS (National Center for Health Statistics). *Advanced Report of Final Mortality Statistics, 1992*. Hyattsville, Maryland: US Department of Health and Human Services, Public Health Service, CDC, 1994 (Monthly Vital Statistics Report, vol. 43, No. 6 suppl.).

Ory, H.W (1981). Ectopic pregnancy and intrauterine contraceptive devices: new perspectives. *Obstetrics and Gynecology*, **57**: 137–144.

Penkava, R., Behling, J. (1979). Ultrasound demonstration of combined ectopic and intrauterine pregnancy. *American Journal of Radiology*, **132**: 1012–1013.

Poland, B.J., Kalousek, D.K. (1986). Embryonic development in ectopic pregnancy. In: *Extrauterine Pregnancy*, (eds, R. Langer, P.P. Iffy), pp. 97–106. PSG Publishing Company, Massachusets.

Reece, E.A., Petrie, R.H., Sirmans, M.F. (1983). Combined intrauterine and extrauterine gestations: a review. *American Journal of Obstetrics and Gynecology*, **146**: 323–330.

Rizk, B., Tan, S.L., Morcos, S., Riddle, A., Brinsden, P., Mason, B., Edwards, R.G. (1991). Heterotopic pregnancies after IVF and ET. *American Journal Obstetrics and Gynecology*, **164**: 161–164.

Rossing, M.A., Daling, J.R., Voigt, L.F., Stergachis, A.S., Weiss, N.S. (1993). Current use of an intrauterine device and risk of tubal pregnancy. *Epidemiology*, **4**: 252–258.

Senterman, M., Jibodh, R, Tulandi, T. (1988). Histopathologic study of amullary and isthmic tubal ectopic pregnancy. *American Journal Obstetrics & Gynecology*, **159**: 939–941.

Sivin, I. (1983). IUDs and ectopic pregnancy. *Studies in Family Planning*, **14**: 57–62.

Stabile, I., Campbell, S., Grudzinskas, J.G. (1989). Ultrasound and circulating placental protein measurements in complications of early pregnancy. *British Journal Obstetrics and Gynecology*, **96**: 1182–1191.

Stabile, I., Grudzinskas, J. G. (1990). Ectopic pregnancy: a review of incidence, etiology and diagnostic aspects. *Obstetrics and Gynecology Survey*, **45**: 335–347.

Snowden, R. (1977). The progestasert and ectopic pregnancy. *British Medical Journal*, **2**: 1600–1601.

Tatum, H.J., Schmidt, F.H (1977). Contraceptive and sterilization practices and extrauterine pregnancy: a realistic perspective. *Fertility and Sterility*, **28**: 407–421.

Tummon, I.S., Whitmore, N.A., Daniel, S.A., Nisker, J.A., Yuzpe, A.A. (1994). Transferring more embryos increases risk of heterotopic pregnancy. *Fertility and Sterility*, **61**(6): 1065–1067.

Vessey, M.P., Doll, R., Johnson, B. (1974). Outcome of pregnancy in women using an intrauterine device. *Lancet*, **1**: 495–498.

Westrom, L., Bengtsson, L., Mardh, P.A. (1981). Incidence, trends and risks of ectopic pregnancy in a population of women. *British Medical Journal*, **282**: 15–22.

Wollen, A. L., Flood, P.R., Sandvei, R., (1984). Morphological changes in tubal mucosa associated with the use of intrauterine contraceptive devices. *British Journal of Obstetrics and Gynaecology*, **91**: 1123–1125.

World Health Organization, Task Force of Intrauterine Devices for Fertility Regulation (1985). A multinational case control study of ectopic pregnancy. *Clinical Reproduction Fertility*, **3**: 131–139.

CHAPTER 2

Clinical presentation of ectopic pregnancy

2.1 Introduction

Ectopic pregnancy remains the great mimic of gynaecology; no other pelvic condition gives rise to more diagnostic errors. The patient may or may not have symptoms pointing to pregnancy. With or without a period of amenorrhoea she typically complains of pelvic pain and irregular vaginal bleeding, but whereas the picture is so characteristic when set down in writing, it is often difficult at the bedside to appreciate the significance of these symptoms. Indeed, only half of the patients with ectopic pregnancy will be correctly diagnosed as having the condition on the basis of clinical features alone (Tuomivaara et al., 1986). The vaginal bleeding is often attributed to a delayed menstrual period or threatened abortion and the pain, if slight, to intestinal colic, whereas tiredness and nausea, if present, are considered to be the ordinary discomforts of a normal pregnancy. In rare cases there are no clinical features to raise suspicion at all. Often the differential diagnosis lies between tubal pregnancy, a normal intrauterine pregnancy with a small ovarian cyst and a threatened, recent or ongoing miscarriage, sometimes in a patient with salpingo-oophoritis.

2.2 Symptomatology

Abdominal pain is the commonest symptom, often present even prior to rupture, but there is little or no correlation between the nature, distribution and radiation of the pain and the final diagnosis. It is entirely a matter of chance how frequent are these attacks of pain prior to tubal abortion or rupture. The pain may be diffuse, bilateral or even contralateral to the ectopic implantation site, thus causing great diagnostic confusion. There may be one or more attacks of very severe pain accompanied by bleeding and shock. The pain may be caused by distension of the tube and separation of the layers of muscle by blood, but severe pain results usually from the presence of blood in the peritoneal cavity. It is unusual for an extrauterine pregnancy to advance beyond six to eight weeks without pain, bleeding or both. Most patients present with amenorrhoea and the last menstrual period (LMP) is often described as lighter than normal. This is not a true period and probably represents withdrawal bleeding secondary to inadequate ovarian steroid levels. One-third of women do not recall the date of their LMP, further contributing to the diagnostic dilemma. Sometimes severe intra-peritoneal bleeding occurs early in the course of ectopic pregnancy, not more than three weeks after a normal menstrual period. The endomet-rium in ectopic pregnancy undergoes a decidual change indistinguishable from that which occurs in normal pregnancy. Irregular vaginal bleeding, which is characteristically scanty and results from sloughing of the decidua, is noted in 50–80% of patients (Stabile and Grudzinskas, 1990). Expulsion of a complete decidual cast is less frequent, often being delayed until there have been several attacks of pain and the pregnancy has been aborted through the tube, or the tube itself ruptured.

In summary, the classical clinical picture of ectopic pregnancy is that of abdominal pain and irregular vaginal bleeding in a woman of reproductive age who may have missed a period. As a rough working rule, if a patient who is a few weeks pregnant complains of a little pain and heavy vaginal bleeding, the pregnancy is probably intrauterine, whereas if she has much pain and little bleeding, she is more likely to have an ectopic pregnancy.

2.3   Clinical examination

The commonest physical sign in women with an ectopic pregnancy is abdominal tenderness, often with rebound. Vaginal bleeding is usual. Bimanual examination should be carried out very gently to avoid rupturing the sac. Approximately half the patients will have an adnexal mass and in two-thirds the uterus appears normal in size; the value of these observations is limited by their subjectivity. On vaginal examin-ation, cervical tenderness is unilateral in half the patients. This sign is often helpful but interpretation depends on consistent examination by the same observer, preferably one who is familiar with the patient's pain threshold. Most patients are afebrile (unless they have a concomitant and usually unrelated infection), thus aiding in the differential diagnosis from pelvic inflammatory disease (PID). An unusual feature is Cullen's sign.

Table 2.1. *Distinction between spontaneous miscarriage and ectopic pregnancy*

Abortion	Ectopic pregnancy
Gradual onset of regular lower abdominal cramps, resembling labour pains	Sudden onset of irregular colicky abdominal pain, sometimes localised to one side
Moderate or heavy vaginal bleeding with clots	Absent or slight vaginal bleeding, often dark
Symptoms of bleeding proportionate to visible blood loss	Symptoms of bleeding and shock greater than visible blood loss
Products of conception seen in vagina	Uterine decidua without chorionic villi only

This is a bluish discoloration around the umbilicus, caused by a considerable quantity of free blood in the peritoneal cavity. Unfortunately none of these physical findings is unique to ectopic pregnancy.

The major gynaecological conditions which mimic ectopic pregnancy are a ruptured or twisted ovarian cyst, acute PID and tubo-ovarian abscess. Each has a typical presentation but none can be unequivocally distinguished from ectopic pregnancy on the basis of clinical features alone. Mittelschmerz characterises a ruptured luteal cyst, but when the pain is on the right, acute appendicitis is a possibility. Typically, in a ruptured luteal cyst, the pain starts in the iliac fossa and tends to decrease with the passage of time. Rarely massive intraperitoneal haemorrhage occurs raising the possibility of tubal abortion. In this case the management is the same (laparoscopy or laparotomy). The sudden onet of abdominal pain followed by repeated episodes of colicky pain with vomiting is typical of a twisted ovarian cyst but exceptions occur. If large enough, the abdomino-pelvic mass may be palpable making the diagnosis easier. Torsion or degeneration of a uterine fibroid may be indistinguishable without ultrasound. Acute salpingitis is the most difficult diagnosis to distinguish from ectopic pregnancy. A vaginal discharge is usual and the temperature may be raised; the pain usually starts in the iliac fossa and is maximal just above the inguinal ligament. Movement of the cervix is extremely painful. Rupture of a tubo-ovarian abscess causes severe pain and shock. A negative pregnancy test (with a detection limit of 25–50 IU/L) virtually excludes ectopic pregnancy (Chapter 3).

Table 2.1 lists the clinical features which may distinguish abortion from ectopic pregnancy. It cannot be overemphasised that exceptions to each point are numerous, and that time should not be wasted on the minutiae of differential diagnosis in the presence of shock.

> **Box 2.1. Clinical presentation of ectopic pregnancy and choice of investigations.**
>
> - Group 1 = acute emergency: laparotomy or laparoscopy
> - Group 2 = at risk: intensive surveillance with serial TVS and hCGs
> - Group 3 = subacute: TVS and/or hCG

2.4   Risk groups

Unless the patient experiences symptoms identical to those in a previous ectopic pregnancy, it is unlikely that individual items in the history and examination will be of value in reaching the diagnosis. It is therefore better to consider the clinical presentation as falling into the three distinct groups (described in Box 2.1). In clinical practice the first step is to identify the group and then act accordingly (Chapter 3).

2.4.1   GROUP 1: ACUTE ABDOMEN

In this group there is evidence of haemoperitoneum with clinical shock (pallor and fainting), falling blood pressure and rising pulse rate following rupture of the tube. These signs correlate well with the amount of blood present in the peritoneal cavity. Rapid intraperitoneal bleeding occurs in less than a quarter of patients with ectopic pregnancy. Blood may irritate the peritoneum by collecting under the diaphragm causing shoulder tip pain or occasionally give rise to the urge to defecate by collecting in the pouch of Douglas. In this emergency situation ectopic pregnancy should be high on the list of differential diagnoses. In practice there is little room for delay in instituting appropriate management as haemorrhagic shock is the commonest reason for the high mortality associated with ectopic pregnancy (May *et al.*, 1976). In one study, over half the women who died from ectopic pregnancy received no treatment and over 80% died from haemorrhage (Atrash *et al.*, 1987).

Apart from a rapid bedside measurement of human chorionic gonadotrophin (hCG) if available, to confirm pregnancy, the emergency situation dictates rapid transfer to the operating theatre for diagnostic laparoscopy or laparotomy. This type of clinical presentation is becoming less common in the western world, possibly because of an increased awareness of ectopic pregnancy by both patients and doctors, as well as earlier referral and the greater availability of diagnostic tests.

2.4.2   GROUP 2: ASYMPTOMATIC HIGH RISK

The second group consists of asymptomatic women at risk of developing ectopic pregnancy for a variety of reasons, such as a past history of ectopic pregnancy (there is a recurrence rate of approximately 10%), previous tubal surgery and subfertile women undergoing assisted conception. Less than 20% of women with ectopic pregnancy fall into this asymptomatic high risk group. Even if one or more of these risk factors is present, intrauterine pregnancy remains the likeliest diagnosis.

Cacciatore and colleagues (1994) screened 225 such symptom-free pregnant women at increased risk for ectopic pregnancy (on the basis of a history of ectopic pregnancy, tubal or pelvic surgery or PID and current users of intrauterine devices) with transvaginal sonography (TVS) and hCG assays. Among 55 (24.4%) women who proved to have an ectopic pregnancy, 46 (84%) of the cases were diagnosed at the initial screening at a median of 37 days of gestation and the rest, at repeated scans, with a false positive rate of 1.2%. Most of the pregnancies were correctly localised by the initial scan at around 5 weeks' gestation and the rest by re-scanning within a few days before complications had occurred. As expected, the initial detection rate was slightly lower in this study than in a previous one from the same group (Cacciatore *et al.*, 1990) which examined sympto-matic patients (84% versus 93%). This is presumably because bleeding within the tube or spillage of blood into the abdominal cavity facilitates detection by TVS in symptomatic patients. Just over 80% of the ectopic pregnancies in the study of Cacciatore *et al.* (1994) could have been diagnosed just by the absence of an intrauterine sac with an hCG level of more than 1000 IU/L, supporting the view that hCG assays supplement TVS in screening for ectopic pregnancy (Grudzinskas and Stabile, 1993). Although intensive surveillance by TVS and serum hCG assay is warranted in this small group of high risk women, it is not known whether reliance on high risk features alone is likely to be cost-effective in the screening of women for ectopic or heterotopic pregnancy.

2.4.3   GROUP 3: SYMPTOMATIC BUT CLINICALLY STABLE

The third and largest group of women with ectopic pregnancy are those with a subacute presentation. If rupture or tubal abortion occur gradually, the symptoms are less dramatic, and the true diagnosis may be missed. There may be a series of small bleeds each accompanied by abdominal pain and faintness. As the circulatory system adjusts the blood pressure, the symptoms improve. This has led to the dictum that any patient with lower abdominal pain and a positive pregnancy test should be considered to have an ectopic pregnancy until proved otherwise. Unless this principle is consistently observed by all practitioners, the non-specific nature of these symptoms will often result in diagnostic delay which may be fatal. For example, an extensive review of maternal deaths from ectopic pregnancy suggested that, in two-thirds of cases, delay in diagnosis and therapy led directly to maternal death and could be ascribed to the attending physician (May *et al.*, 1976). In this group the prospect for early treatment is dependent on maintaining a high index of suspicion and the deployment of a few additional diagnostic tests, the choice of which is dictated by local availability and cost (Chapter 3).

2.5   Point summary

1. Clinical features of ectopic pregnancy are not unique to the condition.

2. Risk factors alone (Group 2) are not a reliable guide to the diagnosis but they may form the basis for a screening test.

3. 75% of patients present with subacute symptoms (Group 3) and 25% or less with an acute abdomen (Group 1).

4. The diagnosis cannot be consistently reached by careful physical examination alone.

5. Investigations are almost always necessary.

6. Morbidity and mortality are directly related to the delay between presentation and treatment.

2.6   References

Atrash, H. K., Friede, A., Hogue, C. J. R. (1987). Ectopic pregnancy mortality in the United States, 1970–1983. *Obstetrics and Gynecology*, **70**: 817–822.

Cacciatore, B., Stenman, U-H., Ylostalo, P. (1990). Diagnosis of ectopic pregnancy by vaginal ultrasonography in combination with a discriminatory serum hCG level of 1000 IU/L (IRP). *British Journal Obstetrics and Gynaecology*, **97**: 904–908.

Cacciatore, B., Stenman, U-H., Ylostalo, P. (1994). Early screening for ectopic pregnancy in high-risk symptom-free women. *Lancet*, **343**: 517–518.

Grudzinskas, J.G., Stabile, I. (1993). Ectopic pregnancy: Are biochemical tests at all useful? *British Journal Obstetrics and Gynaecology*, **100**: 510–511.

May, W.J., Miller, J.B., Greiss, F.C. (1976). Maternal deaths from ectopic pregnancy in the South Atlantic region, 1960 through 1976. *American Journal of Obstetrics and Gynecology*, **132**: 140–147.

Stabile, I., Grudzinskas, J. G. (1990). Ectopic pregnancy: a review of incidence, etiology and diagnostic aspects. *Obstetrics and Gynecology Survey*, **45**: 335–347.

Tuomivaara, L., Kauppila, A., Puolakka, J. (1986). Ectopic pregnancy: an analysis of the etiology, diagnosis and treatment in 552 cases. *Archives of Gynaecology*, **237**: 135–139.

CHAPTER 3

Biochemical diagnosis of ectopic pregnancy

3.1   Introduction

Measurement of human chorionic gonadotrophin (hCG) is the key test in the differential diagnosis of abdominal pain in women of reproductive age. Advances in assay methodology have resulted in the marketing of a wide variety of pregnancy testing kits for home or bedside use. These are summarised in Box 3.1. Measurement of hCG is of particular value in women at high risk for ectopic pregnancy (Group 2) and those with a subacute presentation (Group 3). The current approach to evaluation of the clinically stable patient with a possible ectopic pregnancy also includes an ultrasound examination and occasionally laparoscopy to locate the pregnancy.

The false negative rate of hCG estimation depends on the cut-off level or detection limit of the assay. The lower the detection limit, the fewer the ectopic pregnancies that are missed. State-of-the-art urine hCG assays typically have a detection limit of 25–50 IU/L with false negative rates of less than 2%. Earlier assays with detection limits of 100–500 IU/L should not be used for this indication (Grudzinskas and Stabile, 1993). Whatever the detection limit of the assay, the clinician should maintain a high index of suspicion for ectopic pregnancy even if hCG is undetectable.

Important questions about the use of biochemical tests in ectopic pregnancy remain unresolved. What is the cut-off level most useful in the diagnosis of ectopic pregnancy? Are serial quantitative estimations of greater value than single measurements? Is there is any advantage in multiple biochemical tests? Should they be combined with ultrasound?

3.2   hCG and its subunits

Early diagnosis of pregnancy commonly depends on the detection of hCG in maternal urine or one to two days earlier in blood. The usefulness of an

Box 3.1. Selected urine pregnancy tests for home or bedside use.

Kit	Assay type	Sensitivity	End-point colour	Time (min)
Abbott Testpack	Dye-based sandwich	50 IU/L (1st IRP)	Pink Cross	5
Clear Blue Easy	Dye-based sandwich	50 IU/L (1st IRP)	2 lines if pregnant	3
Clearview hCG	Dye-based sandwich	50 IU/L (1st IRP)	Blue line	5
Concise	Dye-based sandwich	50 IU/L (1st IRP)	Blue line	5–20
Early	Monoclonal immunoassay	50 IU/L	2 lines if pregnant	2–5
EPT	Dye-based twin antibody	35 IU/L	2 lines if pregnant	3
Fact Plus	Sandwich	250 IU/L	Plus sign if pregnant	5
First Response	Dye-based single site	100 IU/L	2 lines if pregnant	3
Tandem Icon II	Dye-based sandwich	20 IU/L (1st IRP)	Blue Spot	7

assay such as hCG to diagnose ectopic pregnancy depends on its clinical sensitivity, i.e. the percentage of ectopic pregnancies with a positive test, and its clinical specificity, i.e. the percentage of non-ectopics with a negative test. Clinical sensitivity and specificity must be distinguished from analytic sensitivity and specificity, i.e. the ability of the test to detect small quantities of the analyte, and only what it purports to measure (Chard, 1986). Ectopic pregnancy may present with serum hCG concentrations that can vary up to four orders of magnitude from as little as 15 IU/L up to 100000 IU/L (DiMarchi *et al.*, 1989).

3.2.1   ASSAY METHODOLOGY

Since the introduction of the first bioassay for hCG (Ascheim and Zondek, 1927), pregnancy testing has become simpler, more sensitive and more rapid (Batzer, 1985). The first generation of immunological hCG tests utilised latex agglutination inhibition methodology. Contamination with blood or excess protein or variations in the concentration of urine gave rise to false positive results. Moreover their sensitivity was low

(500–2000 IU/L), so the tests were positive in only 50% of ectopic pregnancies. Most of these assays could not distinguish between hCG and luteinising hormone (LH). These assays were replaced by radioreceptor assays, which in turn have been largely replaced by enzyme-linked immunoabsorbent assays (ELISAs) and radioimmunoassays (RIAs).

One such rapid single step urine test for hCG (Clearview, Unipath, Bedford) with a detection limit of 50 IU/L has been evaluated in 130 unselected women presenting to an accident and emergency department with lower abdominal pain or abnormal vaginal bleeding and a suspicion of early pregnancy (Kingdom *et al.*, 1991). All 12 women with ectopic pregnancy had a positive test result, although urinary hCG concentrations varied from 191 IU/L to 47 800 IU/L. There was one false positive test. The sensitivity and negative predictive values of this urine pregnancy test were both 100% (95% confidence interval 95.4% to 100%). The additional cost of the test (over cheaper, less sensitive two-stage agglutination tests) is offset by not admitting those patients whose clinical findings are normal and who have a negative urine test result and by reducing the number of women requiring quantitative hCG assays. Moreover, the potential consequences of missing the diagnosis of ectopic pregnancy (increased morbidity, mortality and litigation) make using unreliable pregnancy test kits both dangerous and uneconomical.

Can one rely on a negative hCG result when evaluating suspected ectopic pregnancy? Clearly this depends on the type of test performed and its detection limit. Modern ELISAs which are in widespread use as bedside pregnancy tests utilise monoclonal labelled antibodies. They have a detection limit of 25 IU/L and hence are positive in almost all cases of ectopic pregnancy, a week or more from the expected time of the missed period. There remains, however, a small (probably less than 2%) proportion of cases of ectopic pregnancy in which a sensitive hCG assay (either quantitative RIA or ELISA) is negative (Romero *et al.*, 1985b). This may happen if conception did not occur when expected from the menstrual history (Chard, 1991). The dangers of this observation are tempered by the fact that resorption without rupture often occurs in the hCG-negative ectopic gestation (Lindstedt *et al.*, 1981). Nevertheless, the diagnosis of ectopic pregnancy may still need to be considered when the clinical findings are suggestive of the condition in spite of a negative hCG test result. These women should be assessed by a more experienced clinician or admitted for observation, or both.

Finally, it is worth dispelling the common misconception that if the hCG level is appropriate for the presumed gestational age or if it is greater than 20000 IU/L, then the pregnancy must be intrauterine. On the contrary, tubal pregnancies with hCG levels as high as 90000 IU/L have been reported (Romero *et al.*, 1985a), whereas at least 20% of ectopic pregnancies have hCG levels that are appropriate for gestational age (Braunstein *et al.*, 1978).

3.2.2   ALPHA OR BETA hCG SUBUNITS?

The rate limiting step in the formation of hCG is production of the beta subunit; this then readily combines with the alpha subunit. It is, however, the intact alpha-beta hCG dimer which primarily circulates in the peripheral blood whereas a fragment known as the beta core, consisting of two beta subunit polypeptide chains joined by disulphide bridges, predominates in the urine of pregnant women (Blithe *et al.*, 1988).

The ectopic trophoblast has an impaired ability to synthesise beta but not alpha subunits, such that levels of the free alpha subunit of hCG are higher than those of the free beta subunit in patients with a viable tubal pregnancy (Barnea *et al.*, 1986). It has been suggested that levels of the alpha subunit may reflect an early alteration of trophoblast function at a time when total hCG production is still preserved (L'Hermite-Baleriaux *et al.* 1982). Unfortunately, comparisons of free alpha subunit levels with those of the intact hCG molecule cannot distinguish between spontaneous abortion and ectopic pregnancy.

3.2.3   QUALITATIVE OR QUANTITATIVE TESTS?

Until the last decade, the only quantitative hCG tests available to clinicians were laboratory-based RIAs, the use of which led to delays in instituting appropriate management. These have been replaced by rapid and simple to use dipstick tests which are usually ELISAs; a detailed description of these is beyond the scope of this chapter. Suffice it to say that most of the pregnancy test kits for home or emergency bedside use provide a yes/no answer to the question of whether there is more than a certain level of hCG in the urine, as determined by the detection limit of the test.

Whatever type of test is used, a number of problems and questions face the clinician. The first is deciding between serum and urine hCG testing. While the convenience of urinary testing is obvious, it is often assumed that serum testing is more sensitive; however, the levels of hCG in blood are very similar to those in urine, perhaps because urine is almost always more concentrated (Norman *et al.*, 1988). One exception might be women who receive intravenous fluids (e.g. for rapid bladder filling) prior to transabdominal ultrasound (TAS) before urine is collected. Clinicians should avoid hCG testing on urine samples voided a short while after rapid bladder filling, as false negative results may occur. Unlike latex agglutination inhibition assays, there is no particular advantage in testing early morning urine samples when using RIA or ELISA techniques.

The second question is, how soon after conception can pregnancy be detected by measuring hCG? Using a highly sensitive assay (0.1–0.3 IU/L), maternal circulating hCG is detectable six to seven days after conception, i.e. around the time of implantation (Lenton *et al.*, 1982). When using RIAs with a detection limit of 5 IU/L, hCG is first detectable in serum nine days and in urine 13 days after ovulation (LH surge) in successful *in vitro* fertilisation (IVF) pregnancies (Armstrong *et al.*, 1984). This is equivalent to before the missed period in spontaneous conceptions.

The third problem is that of locating the site of nidation in a woman who is biochemically pregnant. Assuming that hCG levels double every two days (Hamori *et al.*, 1989), there would be a delay of 14 days between biochemical detection of implantation (commonly accepted as an hCG level greater than 10 IU/L) and visualisation of a gestational sac by transvaginal sonography (TVS). Using the abdominal route this interval is even longer (Box 3.2).

As the detection limits of hCG assays have fallen, a fourth problem has emerged. Highly specific and sensitive immunometric assays have revealed the ubiquitous nature of very low hCG levels in non-pregnant (0.02–0.8 IU/L) and even post-menopausal (1–5 IU/L) women (Whittaker *et al.*, 1983). This is rarely a problem in clinical practice as most current pregnancy tests have a sensitivity of 25–50 IU/L (Chard, 1991).

There are various explanations for false positive findings, including the detection of free subunits and the presence of large molecular weight forms of hCG. Other confounding variables include variations in polyclonal antibody specificity for hCG and its beta subunit, cross-reaction with elevated LH levels and unidentified non-specific serum factors. The combined effect of these factors is reflected in the unexpected detection of low levels of hCG in approximately 3% of samples reaching the laboratory (Whittaker, 1988).

To overcome this problem in clinical practice, a single estimation of hCG should be considered diagnostic of pregnancy if it is more than 25 IU/L, or if less than, is seen to double within three days (Jones *et al.*,

1983). The term 'biochemical pregnancy' has been coined to describe those women who have two hCG values of more than 10 IU/L but who go on to apparently normal menstruation.

3.2.4 DISCRIMINATORY hCG ZONE

Kadar *et al*. (1981) were the first to establish that at an hCG level of more than 6500 IU/L (International Reference Preparation; IRP) a gestational sac was visible in 94% of normal pregnancies. The corollary is that if the serum hCG level is more than this in women with suspected ectopic pregnancy and no intrauterine gestational sac can be seen, then an ectopic pregnancy is probably present. They also demonstrated that at an hCG level below 6000 IU/L, the absence of a sac was unhelpful in reaching a diagnosis.

A clinical algorithm based on this 'discriminatory zone', which in this first study was between 6000 IU/L and 6500 IU/L, has been introduced into clinical practice in North America, but has failed to find a place in the UK. There are several possible reasons for this.

First, the threshold level of hCG above which a normal intrauterine gestational sac can be seen ultrasonically is dependent on the resolution of the ultrasound equipment in use, a factor which varies as widely among hospitals in the UK, as it does in the USA. Second, ultrasound examination, which is an integral part of this algorithm, is highly operator dependent. Third, failed pregnancies (both ectopics and spontaneous abortions) typically produce lower hCG levels which increase at a lower rate compared with normal pregnancy. Fourth, values lower than the accepted discriminatory level can still be associated with ectopic pregnancy even if a gestational sac is seen. Fifth, patients with symptoms of pregnancy or its complications may present with hCG values below the accepted discriminatory level. Indeed, in one study only half the patients with ectopic pregnancy at 35–86 days gestation had hCG levels more than 750 IU/L (Second International Standard; IS). This is the cut-off hCG level which allows one to use a vaginosonographic discriminatory hCG zone (DiMarchi *et al*., 1989). Finally, clinicians are aware that results such as those described above cannot be extrapolated from studies carried out in research institutions to smaller district hospitals.

In spite of these reservations, the work of Kadar and colleagues has shown that whatever ultrasound equipment is used, there is an hCG value above which the gestational sac of a normal intrauterine pregnancy is always visible, a level below which it is never detectable and an uncertain zone in between. This deceptively simple principle has revolutionised our

Box 3.2. Published discriminatory hCG levels for the
identification by transabdominal (TAS) and transvaginal (TVS)
ultrasound (U/S) of an intrauterine gestational sac. The level of
the First International Reference Preparation (IRP) of human
chorionic gonadotrophin (hCG) is approximately twice that of
the second International Standard (IS).

Authors	hCG (First IRP)	U/S	hCG (Second IS)
Kadar *et al* (1981)	6500	TAS	
Nyberg *et al* (1985)	3600	TAS	
Romero *et al* (1985a)		TAS	3250
Nyberg *et al* (1987)	1800	TAS	
Cacciatore *et al* (1988)	1800	TAS	
Fossum *et al* (1988)	1398	TVS	914
Goldstein *et al* (1988)		TVS	1025
Nyberg *et al* (1988)		TVS	1000
Bernaschek *et al* (1988)		TVS	300
Bree *et al* (1989)	1000	TVS	
Cacciatore *et al* (1990a)	935	TVS	

understanding of the relationship between sonographic images and hCG
levels in individual patients.

Transvaginal sonography (TVS) has a distinct advantage over TAS, as it
can identify the site of nidation at a lower level of hCG (Box 3.2). The use
of TVS allows a gestational sac to be identified as early as 33 days following
the missed period. The lowest hCG level at which a gestational sac is
consistently visible using TVS is presently 1000 IU/L (IRP) (Cacciatore *et
al.*, 1990b). The sensitivity of beta hCG measurements in combination
with sonographic detection of an adnexal mass in the diagnosis of ectopic
pregnancy is reportedly as high as 96%. The negative predictive value is up
to 92%. Specificity and positive predictive values of 100% have been
reported for the combination of these two tests (Stiller *et al.*, 1989,
Cacciatore *et al.*, 1990a, 1994; Fleischer *et al.*, 1990; Soussis *et al.*, 1991).

3.2.5   SERIAL hCG MEASUREMENTS

Serial quantitative hCG estimations may distinguish normal from abnormal pregnancies. Serum samples taken at least 48 hours apart may indicate

---

Box 3.3. Serial hCGs over 48 hours.

hCG half life < 1.4 days
- Likely diagnosis: spontaneous abortion
- Action: expectant management

1.4–7 days
- Likely diagnosis: abnormal pregnancy
- Action: D&C, proceed to laparoscopy if no villi seen

> 7 days:
- Likely diagnosis: ectopic pregnancy
- Action: surgery

---

levels of hCG that are rising, falling or show no change (Kadar and Romero, 1988).

In patients with rising hCG titres, the rate of increase in hCG (also known as the slope of the log hCG–time regression line) differs between a normal and an abnormal pregnancy. This is the basis for the clinical algorithm introduced by Kadar *et al.* (1981): if hCG increases by less than 66% over 48 hours (equivalent to a doubling time of 2.7 days) then laparoscopy should be performed in clinically stable women with suspected ectopic pregnancies and in whom ultrasound examination is unhelpful (Box 3.3). Some 15% of normal pregnancies will also appear abnormal (false positives) and 13% of ectopic pregnancies would not initially be identified (false negatives) using this approach. Lindblom and colleagues (1989) have refined this concept by plotting the initial hCG value against the rate of change. This so-called hCG score appears to have a useful role in distinguishing normal from pathological pregnancy (but not ectopics from abortions) in patients with hCG levels between 100 IU/L and 4000 IU/L (First IRP) in whom clinical examination and TVS fail to give a clear diagnosis. Hence, normal progression in hCG levels is reassuring in that it confirms trophoblastic growth, but it does not exclude ectopic pregnancy. This is because some ectopic pregnancies with low doubling times for hCG, initially present with normal doubling times, which only later slow down. In addition, abnormal hCG titre progression cannot be used to distinguish between failed intrauterine pregnancy and ectopic pregnancy.

A woman presenting with bleeding prior to six weeks' gestation may cause a diagnostic dilemma. Kadar and Romero (1988) addressed the problem of distinguishing ectopic pregnancy from spontaneous abortion on the basis of falling hCG levels. If serial measurement of hCG over a 48 hour period reveals a fall with a half-life of less than 1.4 days, then a complete abortion is likely and is best managed expectantly. If the half life is greater than seven days then an ectopic pregnancy is likely. Thus contrary to popular belief, falling hCG levels are not synonymous with spontaneous abortion; the half-life of hCG levels can be used to distinguish abortion from an ectopic pregnancy. A plateau in hCG levels, defined as an hCG doubling time of seven days or more, is also highly suggestive of ectopic pregnancy (Kadar and Romero, 1988).

3.2.6   LIMITATIONS OF hCG FOR THE DIAGNOSIS OF ECTOPIC GESTATION

There are a number of limitations to the use of hCG as a screening test for ectopic pregnancy in a low risk population. First, hormone secretion by an ectopically implanted trophoblast is generally lower than that of an intrauterine trophoblast. There are two major reasons for this: poor vascular support in the fallopian tube and inherently diminished hormonal function. There is no pattern of hormone production that unambiguously identifies ectopic pregnancy.

Second, although the steep rise in hormone levels in early pregnancy makes it possible to use hormone concentration (not only hCG but also human placental lactogen (hPL) and Schwangerschafts protein 1 (SP1)) to predict gestational age, once the pregnancy begins to fail the pattern of hCG production, although diminished, is inconsistent. Moreover, the half-life of hCG after spontaneous miscarriage is between three days and seven days (Schwartz and DiPietro, 1980); thus the pregnancy might be thought to be ongoing when in fact the trophoblast is degenerating.

Third, the interpretation of quantitative biochemical data is dependent on an accurate knowledge of the duration of amenorrhoea, which is missing in at least one-third of patients with ectopic pregnancy (Stabile and Grudzinskas, 1990). Together with irregular vaginal bleeding, this problem limits the sole use of urine or serum hCG measurement in the management of suspected ectopic pregnancy.

Fourth, the use of serial quantitative estimations involves waiting for at least 48 hours during which time the ectopic may rupture. Moreover, the cost of screening an unselected population for ectopic pregnancy is high as a 24-hour laboratory service is required. In many cases an ultrasound examination is required to locate the pregnancy, further adding to the cost considerations.

Fifth, comparison of pregnancy tests between laboratories should take into account which standard was used to calibrate the test. The Second International Standard (IS) developed by the World Health Organization

(WHO) is contaminated by free alpha and beta subunits and when used in immunoassays is equivalent to approximately half of the more recent and purer standard known as the International Reference Preparation (IRP). This is particularly important when correlating quantitative hCG levels with sonographic findings (Section 3.2.4).

Finally, although there is now consensus about the lowest hCG value above which the gestational sac of an intrauterine pregnancy can always be detected using ultrasound (currently approximately 1000 IU/L (Box 3.2), the predictive value for ectopic pregnancy of an hCG above this level with no identifiable sac is as yet uncertain.

3.2.7   hCG REGRESSION

It may be necessary, under certain circumstances, to evaluate the rate of fall of hCG, e.g. for identification of continued trophoblastic growth after conservative surgical resection or medical treatment with chemotherapeutic agents, as well as the follow-up of those women in whom a very early ectopic pregnancy is being monitored expectantly without treatment. In each of these cases, persistence of a viable trophoblast would be expected to lengthen the half-life of hCG. Another way of measuring hCG regression is by plotting the follow-up values as a percentage of the pre-treatment hCG level, using nomograms for the index time period (Holtz, 1983).

3.3   Other biochemical tests

Other pregnancy parameters have been examined as possible ancillary tests in suspected ectopic pregnancy. None of these has received widespread acceptance in clinical practice so only a brief description is given here. Further details of these research methods may be found in Stabile (1988).

3.3.1   SCHWANGERSCHAFTSPROTEIN 1 (SP1)

SP1 is a trophoblast glycoprotein that appears in the maternal circulation shortly after implantation. It is potentially a useful marker of pregnancy, but quantitative estimations are no better than hCG in distinguishing between intra- and extrauterine pregnancy (Braunstein and Asch, 1983).

3.3.2   PREGNANCY-ASSOCIATED PLASMA PROTEIN A (PAPP-A)

PAPP-A is another trophoblastic glycoprotein; its levels are low or undetectable in most cases of ectopic pregnancy. Immunohistochemical (Tornehave *et al.*, 1986) and cell explant experiments (Stabile, 1988) have confirmed that PAPP-A synthesis by the trophoblast is severely and selectively compromised in ectopic gestation. It cannot be detected in normal pregnancy until six to seven weeks' gestation and so the clinical value of these observations is limited.

3.3.3   HUMAN PLACENTAL LACTOGEN (HPL)

HPL can be detected in the maternal circulation from six weeks. HPL values are often normal in an ectopic pregnancy, even when the levels of hCG or SP1 are abnormal (Braunstein and Asch, 1983).

3.3.4   CORPUS LUTEUM: PROGESTERONE, OESTRADIOL AND RELAXIN

It has been assumed that a very early ectopic gestation has normal endocrine function; however progesterone levels may be low in asymptomatic women with ectopic pregnancy 14–21 days after spontaneous conception despite normal hCG levels (Lower *et al.*, 1992). The sensitivity of a serum progesterone value below 15 ng/ml to distinguish between normal and ectopic pregnancies is approximately 80% (Buck *et al.*, 1988) with false positive rates of around 10% (Stovall *et al.*, 1989). In the patient clinically suspected of having an ectopic pregnancy, a progesterone level below 20 ng/mL suggests early pregnancy failure regardless of the gestational age (Sauer *et al.*, 1989). At a progesterone cut-off level of 9.4 ng/mL the specificity for abnormal pregnancy is in excess of 95% (Hahlin *et al.* 1990); however the problem in clinical practice is to distinguish spontaneous abortion from ectopic pregnancy. The finding of low progesterone levels does not help with this distinction (Gelder *et al.*, 1991).

Eighty per cent of women with ectopic pregnancy have oestradiol levels below the tenth centile of the normal range (Hubinont *et al.*, 1987) except when a live embryo is found (Jouppila *et al.*, 1980). Relaxin levels are higher in a complicated than in a normal early pregnancy but cannot be used to distinguish between an ectopic pregnancy and a spontaneous abortion (Seeger *et al.*, 1988).

3.3.5   ENDOMETRIAL AND DECIDUAL PROTEINS: PP12, PP14

The two major proteins synthesised by the human endometrium, progesterone dependent endometrial protein (PEP, also known as placental protein 14, PP14) and insulin-like growth factor binding protein-1 (IGFBP-1, also known as placental protein 12, PP12), have recently emerged as possible biochemical markers for ectopic pregnancy. IGFBP-1 measurements are of limited clinical value in this situation because of the overlap in levels between a failed intrauterine pregnancy and an ectopic pregnancy (Stabile *et al.*, 1989a, 1990). Decidual synthesis of IGFBP-1 does not seem to depend on anatomical contact between decidua and trophoblast. By contrast PP14, which is derived mainly from the glandular epithelium, is depressed in patients with an ectopic pregnancy and appears to distinguish between an ectopic gestation and a spontaneous abortion (Ruge *et al.*, 1991; Stabile *et al.*, 1994).

3.3.6   FETAL PROTEINS: ALPHAFETOPROTEIN (AFP)

Normal or elevated AFP levels are observed in women with a live ectopic pregnancy, although the clinical value of these observations is limited because only 15–20% of ectopic pregnancies fall into this category (Stabile *et al.*, 1989b,c).

3.3.7   ENZYMES: ALPHA AMYLASE, RENIN AND PRORENIN

Case reports have documented elevated serum and peritoneal fluid amylase levels in ruptured ectopic pregnancy (Fledge, 1966). This has not been confirmed by larger studies (Hannon and Guzick, 1985). By contrast, evaluation of the enzymes prorenin and active renin by Meunier *et al.* (1991) has given encouraging results. The combination of low hCG (less than 15000 IU/L) and low active renin (less than 30 pg/mL) had a predictive value positive of 75% and a predictive value negative of 97% for ectopic pregnancy.

3.4   Do I have an ectopic pregnancy?: A Bayesian analytic approach

In recent years there has been a resurgence of interest in the process of clinical reasoning. We present here a brief exposition of the probabilistic interpretation of the results of diagnostic tests in suspected ectopic pregnancy by means of Bayesian analysis. This approach combines both the physician's diagnostic hypotheses before testing and the test result itself. It is described in terms of probabilities, i.e. the relative frequency with which an event is likely to occur. Clearly such a probability can never be known with certainty and is usually estimated on the basis of personal experience with similar cases and from a survey of the literature.

A prior probability is a belief about the likelihood of a diagnostic hypothesis (for example ectopic pregnancy) given all information collected up to a certain point. It thus represents the belief before testing and is taken to be equivalent to the prevalence of the disease in a group of patients similar to that being tested. A posterior probability represents the revised belief in the likelihood of the diagnosis after interpreting the test result. Test characteristics are defined as conditional probabilities which describe the relative frequency with which a given result occurs in a given disease and in all other diagnoses of potential interest.

Bayesian analysis can be used in medical diagnosis provided two assumptions hold true. The first is that the diagnostic hypotheses under consideration (for example normal pregnancy, spontaneous abortion, ectopic pregnancy, pelvic inflammatory disease and ovarian cyst) are mutually exclusive and include the true diagnosis. The second is that the result of each diagnostic test (in this example we consider hCG and ultrasound) are independent of the results of all other tests.

The simplest form of Bayes' rule is:

$$\text{pHypothesis/Evidence} = \frac{\text{pHypothesis} \times \text{pEvidence/Hypothesis}}{\text{pEvidence}}$$

The ratio defines whether the evidence (in this case biochemical, sonographic etc.) is more likely to be observed when the hypothesis is true than for a randomly selected patient. For example, consider the probability that a woman is pregnant given that she has amenorrhoea. In that case the ratio will be greater than one because amenorrhoea is more likely to occur in pregnant women than in a randomly selected group of women.

We have applied Bayesian analysis to numerical data extracted from Stabile *et al.* (1988, 1989d) and Nyberg *et al.* (1991). In a group of women who believed they were pregnant and who presented with either abdominal pain, vaginal bleeding or both and in whom ectopic pregnancy was suspected clinically, a positive hCG result (more than 25 IU/L) increased the likelihood of ectopic pregnancy from 25% to 60%. In the

Box 3.4. Bayesian analysis of ultrasound data in suspected ectopic pregnancy.

Suspected ectopic pregnancy	Prior probability	Any abnormal U/S finding	Positive result	Posterior probability
Ectopic	0.25	0.65	0.163/0.468	0.335
No ectopic	0.75	0.43	0.323/0.486	0.665

Box 3.5. Bayesian analysis of hCG data in suspected ectopic pregnancy.

Suspected ectopic pregnancy	Prior probability	hCG > 25IU/L	Positive result	Posterior probability
Ectopic	0.25	1.0	0.25/0.393	0.636
No ectopic	0.75	0.19	0.143/0.393	0.364

same group of women with suspected ectopic pregnancy, any abnormal abdominal ultrasound finding (defined here as free fluid in the pouch of Douglas, endometrial thickness of more than 10 mm, uterine area less than 20 cm, adnexal mass volume of more than 10 cm) increased the likelihood of ectopic pregnancy from 25% to 33% (Boxes 3.4 and 3.5).

3.5   Practical considerations

We have shown that most women clinically suspected of having an ectopic pregnancy are in fact not pregnant at all (Stabile *et al.*, 1988). The above Bayesian analysis has demonstrated that, in a group of women in whom ectopic pregnancy is suspected, a positive hCG result (more than 25 IU/L) increases the likelihood of ectopic pregnancy from 25% to 60%, whereas an abnormal finding on abdominal ultrasound (except a live fetal pole in the adnexa) increases the likelihood only marginally from 25% to 33%. Thus if TVS is unavailable, evaluation of these patients should begin with an hCG test. If the test is negative, ectopic pregnancy is most unlikely. If the test is positive, ultrasound is indicated to locate the site of nidation. This assumes that the standard of ultrasound is such that the results can be relied upon. This is not necessarily true for all units; it can be argued that if a patient presents with an acute abdomen (Group 1) or with high risk features of ectopic gestation (Group 2) and is shown to be pregnant, that in itself may be sufficient indication for laparoscopy.

The biochemical diagnosis of an ectopic pregnancy is not straight-forward. There are several problems. First, ectopic pregnancy is not a homogeneous condition; there are differences in clinical presentation, viability and gestational age at presentation. Second, if the early ectopic pregnancy is functioning normally, biochemical tests will be of no diagnostic value. Third, as diagnostic hypotheses are dependent on disease prevalence, the ability of biochemical tests to predict viability or to screen asymptomatic women for either an ectopic pregnancy or an abortion (as determined in the published literature), cannot be extrapo-lated to the symptomatic population in which exclusion of an ectopic pregnancy is a genuine problem. Equally, the results of a Bayesian analysis such as that in Box 3.5 cannot be applied to a different study population (for example asymptomatic women).

These factors combine to make the diagnosis more difficult as the test which can be applied in one situation may be less useful in another. The most sensible (and cost effective) approach is to select biochemical tests depending on the clinical situation. For example, in the acute situation (Group 1) in which the tube has ruptured, both luteal and trophoblastic function are generally normal. The only test needed is a simple qualitative hCG measurement to confirm that the acute abdomen is due to a complication of pregnancy. By contrast, women presenting with subacute symptoms (Group 3 patients) generally have depressed protein and steroid secretion; a situation that can only be identified by sensitive quantitative hCG assays. Progesterone estimations may help to distin-guish between a viable intrauterine pregnancy and a pathological pregnancy, whether intra- or extrauterine. Distinguishing between an ectopic pregnancy and a spontaneous abortion in pregnant Groups 2 and 3 patients is best achieved by diagnostic ultrasound (Chapter 4).

3.6   Point summary

1. Hormone levels produced by the ectopically implanted trophoblast are generally lower than those of an intrauterine pregnancy.

2. There is no hormonal profile that is pathognomonic of an ectopic pregnancy.

3. hCG can be used as a sensitive marker for trophoblastic tissue located either within or outside the uterus.

4. As compared with normal intrauterine pregnancies, patients with ectopic pregnancies have lower hCG values which may either decline slowly, have a slow subnormal rise or plateau.

5. If the serum hCG is rising, the likelihood that the pregnancy is extrauterine rather than intrauterine increases as the hCG doubling time increases.

6. Most women with an hCG half-life greater than seven days (plateau) have an ectopic pregnancy, whereas spontaneous abortion is more likely when the half-life is less than 1.4 days.

7. If serial hCG measurements are not available, distinguishing between ectopic pregnancy and spontaneous abortion in pregnant women is probably best achieved by ultrasound.

8. A single progesterone value does not reliably predict the presence or absence of an ectopic pregnancy.

3.7   References

Armstrong, E.G., Ehrlich, P.H., Birken, S. (1984). Use of a highly sensitive and specific immunoradiometric assay for detection of hCG in urine of normal, non-pregnant and pregnant individuals. *Journal of Clinical Endocrinological Metabolism*, **59**: 867–874.

Ascheim, S., Zondek, B. (1927). Anterior pituitary hormone and ovarian hormone in the urine of pregnant women. *Klinik Wochenschr*, **6**, 1322–1326.

Barnea, E.R., Oelsner, G., Benveniste, R. (1986). Progesterone, oestradiol and alpha human chorionic gonadotropin secretion in patients with ectopic pregnancy. *Journal of Clinical Endocrinology and Metabolism*, **62**: 529–534.

Batzer, F.R. (1985). Guidelines for choosing a pregnancy test. *Contemporary Obstetrics and Gynecology*, **26** (Suppl.): 37–40.

Bernaschek, G., Rudelstorfer, R., Csaicsich, P. (1988). Vaginal sonography versus serum hCG in early detection of pregnancy. *American Journal of Obstetrics and Gynecology*, **158**: 608–612.

Blithe, D.L., Akar, A.H., Wehmann, R.E., Nisula, B.C. (1988). Purification of beta-core fragment from pregnancy urine and demonstration that its carbohydrate moieties differ from those of native human chorionic gonadotropin-beta. *Endocrinology*, **122**(1): 173–180.

Braunstein, G.D., Asch, R.H. (1983). Predictive value analysis of measurements of hCG, pregnancy specific beta-l-glycoprotein, placental lactogen and cystine aminopeptidase for the diagnosis of ectopic pregnancy. *Fertility and Sterility*, **39**, 62–67.

Braunstein, G.D., Karow, W.G., Gentry, W.C. (1978). First trimester chorionic gonadotropin measurement as an aid in the diagnosis of early pregnancy disorder. *American Journal of Obstetrics and Gynecology*, **131**: 25–32.

Bree, L.R., Edwards, M., Bohm Velez, M., Beyler, S., Roberts, J., Mendelson, A.B. (1989). Transvaginal sonography in the evaluation of normal early pregnancy: correlation with hCG levels. *American Journal of Radiology*, **153**: 75–79.

Buck, R.H., Joubert, S.M., Norman, R.J. (1988). Serum progesterone in the diagnosis of ectopic pregnancy: a valuable diagnostic test? *Fertility and Sterility*, **50**, 752–755.

Cacciatore, B., Stenman, U-H., Ylostalo, P. (1990a) Diagnosis of ectopic pregnancy by vaginal ultrasonography in combination with a discriminatory serum hCG level of 1000 IU/l (IRP). *British Journal Obstetrics and Gynaecology*, **97**, 904–908.

Cacciatore, B., Stenman, U-H., Ylostalo, P. (1994). Early screening for ectopic pregnancy in high-risk symptom-free women. *Lancet*, **343**, 517–518.

Cacciatore, B., Tiitinen, A., Stenman, D.H., Ylostalo, P. (1990b). Normal early pregnancy: serum hCG levels and vaginal ultrasonography findings. *British Journal of Obstetrics and Gynaecology*, **97**, 899–903.

Cacciatore, B., Ylostalo, P., Stenman U.H., Widholm, O. (1988). Suspected ectopic pregnancy: ultrasound findings and hCG levels assessed by an immunofluorometric assay. *British Journal of Obstetrics and Gynaecology*, **95**: 497–502.

Chard, T. (1986). *An Introduction to Radioimmunoassay and Related Techniques.* New York, Elsevier Biomedical.

Chard, T. (1991). Frequency of implantation of early pregnancy loss in natural cycles. In: *Balliere's Clinical Obstetrics and Gynaecology*, pp. 179–189. Balliere-Tindall, London.

DiMarchi, J. M., Josas, T. S., Hale, R. W. (1989). What is the significance of hCG value in ectopic pregnancy? *Obstetrics and Gynecology*, **74**, 851–855.

Fledge, J.B. (1966). Ruptured tubal pregnancy with elevated serum amylase levels. *Archives of Surgery (Chicago)*, **92**, 397–398.

Fleischer, A.C., Pennell, R.G., McKee, M.S., Worrell, J.A., Keefe, B., Herbert, C.M., Hill, G.A., Cartwright, P.S., Keeple, D.M. (1990).

Ectopic pregnancy: features at transvaginal sonography. *Radiology*, **174**: 375–378.

Fossum, G.T., Davajan, V., Kletzky, O.A. (1988). Early detection of pregnancy with transvaginal ultrasound. *Fertility and Sterility* **49**: 788–791.

Gelder, M.S., Boots, L.R., Younger, J.B. (1991). Use of a single random progesterone value as a diagnostic aid for ectopic pregnancy. *Fertility and Sterility*, **55**, 497–500.

Goldstein, S.R., Snyder, J.R., Watson, C., Danon, M. (1988). Very early pregnancy detection with endovaginal ultrasound. *Obstetrics and Gynecology*, **72**, 200–204.

Grudzinskas, J.G., Stabile, I. (1993). Ectopic pregnancy: are biochemical tests at all useful? *British Journal of Obstetrics and Gynaecology*, **100**, 510–511.

Hahlin, M., Wallin, A., Sjoblom, P., Lindblom, B. (1990). Single progesterone assay for early recognition of abnormal pregnancy. *Human Reproduction*, **5**, 622–626.

Hamori, M., Stuckensen, J. A., Rumpf, D. (1989). Early pregnancy wastage following late implantation of embryos after IVF/ET. *Human Reproduction*, **4**: 714–717.

Hannon, Z. J., Guzick, D.S. (1985). Tubal pregnancy: significance of serum and peritoneal fluid and alpha amylase. *Obstetrics and Gynecology*, **66**: 395–397.

Holtz, G. (1983). Human chorionic gonadotropin regression following conservative surgical management of tubal pregnancy. *American Journal of Obstetrics and Gynecology*, **147**: 347–350.

Hubinont, C. H., Thomas, C., Schwers, J. F. (1987). Luteal function in ectopic pregnancy. *American Journal of Obstetrics and Gynecology*, **156**: 669–673.

Jones, H.W., Acosta, A.A., Andrews, M.C. (1983). What is pregnancy? A question for IVF. *Fertility and Sterility*, **40**: 728–733.

Jouppila, P., Huhtaniemi, I., Tapanainen, J. (1980). Early pregnancy failure: study by ultrasonic and hormonal methods. *Obstetrics and Gynecology*, **55**: 42–47.

Kadar, N., DeVore, G., Romero, R. (1981). Discriminatory hCG zone: its use in the sonographic evaluation for ectopic pregnancy. *Obstetrics and Gynecology*, **58**: 156–161.

Kadar, N., Romero, R. (1988). Further observations on serial hCG patterns in ectopic pregnancy and abortions. *Fertility and Sterility*, **50**: 367–370.

Kingdom, J.C., Kelly, T., MacLean, A.B., McAllister, E.J. (1991). Rapid one step urine pregnancy test for hCG in evaluating suspected complications of early pregnancy. *British Medical Journal*, **302**(6788): 1308–1311.

L'Hermite-Baleriaux, A.M., VanExter, C., Deville, J.L. (1982). Alteration of free hCG subunits secretion in ectopic pregnancy. *Acta Endocrinologica*, **100**, 109–113.

Lenton, E.A., Neal, L.M., Sulaimen, R. (1982). Plasma concentration of hCG from the time of implantation until the second week of pregnancy. *Fertility and Sterility*, **37**, 773–778.

Lindblom, B., Hahlin, M., Sjoblom, P. (1989). Serial hCG determinations by fluoroimmunoassay for differentiation between intrauterine and ectopic gestation. *American Journal of Obstetrics and Gynecology*, **161**, 397–400.

Lindstedt, G., Janson, P.O., Thorburn, J. (1981). Sensitivity of serum chorionic gonadotropin for ectopic pregnancy. *Lancet*: 781–782.

Lower, A.M., Yovich, J.L., Hancock, C., Grudzinskas, J.G. (1992). Is luteal function maintained by factors other than hCG in early pregnancy? *British Journal of Obstetrics and Gynaecology*, **99**: 704.

Meunier, K., Guichard, A., Mignot, T.M., Zorn, J.R., Maria, B., Cedard, L. (1991). Predictive value of active renin assay for the diagnosis of ectopic pregnancy. *Fertility and Sterility*, **55**: 432–435.

Norman, R.J., Buck, R.H., Rom, L. (1988). Blood or urine measurement of hCG for detection of ectopic pregnancy? A comparative study of quantitative and qualitative methods in both fluids. *Obstetrics and Gynecology*, **71**, 315–318.

Nyberg, D.A., Filly, R.A., Laing, F.C., Mack, L.A., Zarutskie, P.W. (1987). Ectopic pregnancy. Diagnosis by sonography correlated with quantitative hCG levels. *Journal of Ultrasound Medicine*, **6**: 145–150.

Nyberg, D.A., Filly, R.A., Mahony, B.S., Monroe, S., Laing, F.C., Jeffrey, R.B. Jr. (1985). Early gestation: correlation of hCG levels and sonographic identification. *American Journal of Roentgenology*, **144**: 951–954.

Nyberg, D.A., Hughes, M.P., Mack, L., Wang, K.W. (1991). Extrauterine findings of ectopic pregnancy at transvaginal ultrasound: importance of echogenic fluid. *Radiology*, **178**: 823–826.

Nyberg, D.A., Mack, L.A., Laing, F.C., Jeffrey, R.B. (1988). Early pregnancy complications: endovaginal sonographic findings correlated with human chorionic gonadotrophin levels. *Radiology*, **167**: 619–622.

Romero, R., Kadar, N., Copel, J.A. (1985a). The effect of different human chorionic gonadotropin assay sensitivity on screening for ectopic pregnancy. *American Journal of Obstetrics and Gynecology*, **153**: 72–77.

Romero, R., Kadar, N., Jeanty, P. (1985b). The diagnosis of ectopic pregnancy: the value of the hCG discriminatory zone. *Obstetrics and Gynecology*, **66**: 357–360.

Ruge, S., Sorensen, S., Pedersen, J.F., Lange, A.P., Brjalsen, I., Bohn, H. (1991). Secretory endometrial protein PP14 in women with early pregnancy bleeding. *Human Reproduction*, **6**: 885–888.

Sauer, M.V., Sinosich, M.J., Yeko, T.R. (1989). Predictive value of a single

PAPP-A or progesterone in the diagnosis of abnormal pregnancy. *Human Reproduction*, **4**: 331–334.

Schwartz, R.O. and DiPietro, D.L. (1980). Beta hCG as a diagnostic aid for suspected ectopic pregnancy. *Obstetrics and Gynecology*, **56**: 197–203.

Seeger, H., Zwirner, M., Voelter, W., Lippert, TH. (1988). Relaxin and human chorionic gonadotropin concentrations in blood serum during the first trimester of normal and pathological pregnancy. *Gynecologic and Obstetric Investigation*, **25**(3): 209–212.

Soussis, I., Dimitri, E.S., Oskarsson, T., Margara, R., Winston, R. (1991). Diagnosis of ectopic pregnancy by vaginal ultrasonography in combination with a discriminatory serum hCG level of 1000 IU/L. *British Journal of Obstetrics and Gynaecology*, **98**: 223.

Stabile, I. (1988). *Pregnancy associated plasma protein A in complications of early pregnancy with particular reference to ectopic gestation*. Ph.D. Thesis, University of London.

Stabile, I., Grudzinskas, J.G. (1990). Ectopic pregnancy: a review of incidence, etiology and diagnostic aspects. *Obstetrical and Gynecological Survey*, **45**, 335–347.

Stabile, I., Campbell, S., Grudzinskas, J.G. (1988). Can ultrasound reliably diagnose ectopic pregnancy? *British Journal of Obstetrics and Gynaecology*, **95**: 1247–1252.

Stabile, I., Campbell, S., Grudzinskas, J.G. (1989d). Ultrasound and circulating placental protein measurements in complications of early pregnancy. *British Journal of Obstetrics and Gynaecology*, **96**: 1182–1191.

Stabile, I., Chard, T., Grudzinskas, J.G. (1994). Circulating pregnancy protein 14 levels in ectopic pregnancy. *British Journal of Obstetrics and Gynaecology*, **101**: 762–764.

Stabile, I., Howell, R., Teisner, B., Chard, T., Grudzinskas, J. G. (1989a). Circulating levels of PP12 in complications of first trimester pregnancy. *Archives of Gynecology and Obstetrics*, **246**: 201–206.

Stabile, I., Olajide, F., Chard, T., Grudzinskas, J.G. (1989b). Maternal serum alphafetoprotein levels in anembryonic pregnancy. *Human Reproduction*, **4**: 204–205.

Stabile, I., Olajide, F., Chard, T., Grudzinskas, J.G. (1989c). Maternal serum alphafetoprotein levels in ectopic pregnancy. *Human Reproduction*, **4**, 835–836.

Stabile, I., Teisner, B., Chard, T., Grudzinskas, J. G. (1990). Circulating levels of PP12 in ectopic pregnancy. *Archives of Gynecology and Obstetrics*, **247**: 149–153.

Stiller, R.J., de Regt, R.H., Blair, E. (1989). Transvaginal sonography in patients at risk for ectopic pregnancy. *American Journal of Obstetrics and Gynecology*, **161**: 930–933.

Stovall, T.G., Ling, F.W., Cope, B.J. (1989). Preventing ruptured ectopic pregnancy with a single serum progesterone. *American Journal of Obstetrics and Gynecology*, **160**: 1425–1431.

Tornehave, D., Chemnitz, J., Westergaard, J.G. (1986). Placental proteins in peripheral blood and tissues of ectopic pregnancies. *Gynecologic and Obstetric Investigation*, **23**: 97–102.

Whittaker, P.G. (1988). Recognition of early pregnancy hCG. In *Implantation: Biological and Clinical Aspects* eds. M.G. Chapman, J.G. Grudzinskas, T. Chard, pp. 33–40. Springer-Verlag, London.

Whittaker, P.G., Taylor, A., Lind, T. (1983). Unsuspected pregnancy loss in healthy women. *Lancet*, 1126–1127.

CHAPTER 4

Ultrasound diagnosis of ectopic pregnancy

4.1 Introduction

The role of ultrasonography in suspected ectopic gestation is to localise the pregnancy. If intrauterine, ectopic pregnancy is excluded as the combination of intra- and extrauterine pregnancy (heterotopic pregnancy) is exceedingly rare in spontaneous conceptions; however, failed intrauterine pregnancy (missed, complete and incomplete abortion) may be indistinguishable from ectopic pregnancy. The introduction of transvaginal sonography (TVS) using high frequency transducers has proved a major advance in this area. Even with TVS, however, an ectopic embryo/fetus is seen in only 20% of cases (DeCrespigny, 1988). In the remainder there may or may not be other sonographic features which assist with the diagnosis. The predictive value of the vaginosonographic parameters of ectopic pregnancy is still uncertain; better images should not be equated with more accurate diagnosis (Bateman et al, 1990; Russell *et al.*, 1993).

4.2 Comparison between abdominal and vaginal ultrasound

The major advantage of TVS over transabdominal sonography (TAS) is that TVS can diagnose normal and failed intrauterine pregnancy at least one week earlier. Most comparisons of TVS and TAS in women with abdominal pain have been retrospective (Lande *et al.*, 1988), or not designed to compare the two techniques (Coleman *et al.*, 1988; Lande *et al.*, 1988), or failed to correlate sonographic findings with surgical outcome in the whole study group (Coleman *et al.*, 1988; Lande *et al.*, 1988; Liebman *et al.*, 1988; Mendelson *et al.*, 1988). Andolf and

Jorgensen (1990) performed a prospective study of 85 patients who underwent TAS and TVS 24 hours before elective surgery for a variety of gynaecological diseases. In spite of better image quality, TVS was not superior to TAS, particularly in the evaluation of large ovarian cysts and fibroids.

Many studies claim to compare TVS and TAS in the diagnosis of early pregnancy failure (for review see Stabile, 1992). There are significant differences in the criteria for entry into these studies. Most are retrospective and examinations are often performed by multiple operators, sometimes submitting hard copy images for later interpretation. Without clinical, surgical or pathological follow-up (as occurred in some of these studies), it is impossible to determine false negative rates. Moreover, if the aim of a study is to evaluate the clinical benefit of a diagnostic test, then it is important that the patient group studied should represent a true diagnostic problem, rather than being a simple exercise in data collection.

4.3 Sonographic features of intrauterine pregnancy

The sonographic features of a normal intrauterine pregnancy are summarised in Box 4.1. Pregnancy can be diagnosed ultrasonically by demonstrating an intrauterine gestation sac (Figure 4.1). This is consistently possible using TAS from six weeks amenorrhea onwards, although Yeh *et al.* (1986) reported finding focal echogenic thickening of the endometrium as early as 3.5 weeks from the last menstrual period (LMP) using TAS. The consistent demonstration of a gestation sac within the uterus from 4.5 weeks onwards is possible with TVS (Jain *et al.*, 1988). It is important to distinguish between the consistent observation of a feature (the discriminatory level) and its earliest detection (the threshold level). Failure to do so accounts for the variation in gestational age at which ultrasound features are reported. For example, a gestation sac (mean diameter of 2 mm) was identified in only two of eight patients at human chorionic gonadotrophin (hCG) values between 50 IU/L and 280 IU/L (second IS) two days after the missed period (the threshold level), whereas a gestation sac was always seen (discriminatory level) at hCG levels greater than 300 IU/L (Bernaschek *et al.*, 1988). Each ultrasound department must determine their own threshold and discriminatory levels, on the basis of the

---

Box 4.1. Transvaginal ultrasound features of intrauterine pregnancy.

1. Day 30: earliest detectable gestation sac (diameter 2 mm)
2. Days 33–35:
   - Consistently detectable eccentric intrauterine sac with asymmetrical trophoblast ring
   - Double echogenic wall appearance: decidua capsularis and parietalis (also seen in up to 30% of ectopic pregnancy)
3. Days 38–40: earliest embryonic heart activity and yolk sac detected
4. Day 46: consistent detection of embryonic echoes with visible heart motion

---

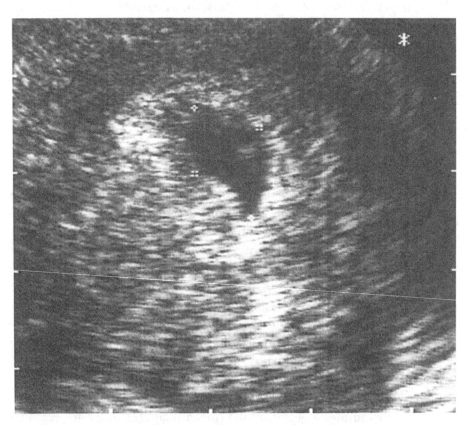

Figure 4.1 Transvaginal ultrasound at five weeks after embryo transfer depicting an eccentrically located intrauterine gestation sac with asymmetrical trophoblast ring (normal intrauterine pregnancy).

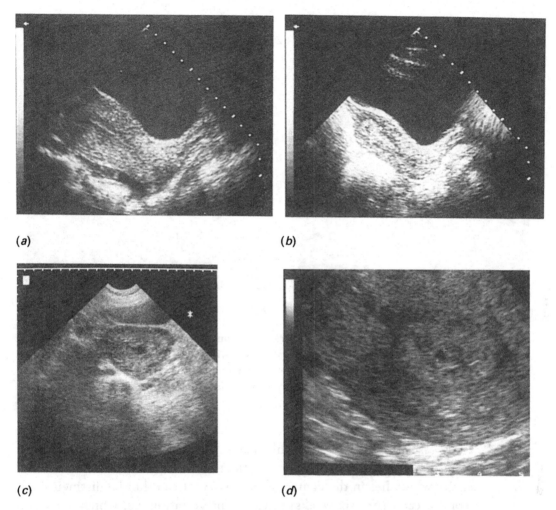

(a)   *(b)*

(c)   *(d)*

Figure 4.2 *(a)* Transabdominal ultrasound: longitudinal section of normal non-pregnant uterus depicting clear endometrial interface and a little fluid in the pouch of Douglas. *(b)* Transabdominal ultrasound: longitudinal section of uterus containing thickened, irregular hyperplastic endometrium. The adnexa contained an ectopic pregnancy (not shown). *(c)* Transabdominal ultrasound: transverse section of uterus containing a pseudogestation sac. *(d)* Transvaginal ultrasound: transverse section of uterus containing normal intrauterine pregnancy at five weeks gestation.

experience of their staff, the resolution of their equipment and an audit of their results.

The definitive diagnosis of a viable intrauterine pregnancy must include the demonstration of fetal heart activity within the uterine gestation sac. This is particularly important when TAS is being used to evaluate a suspected ectopic pregnancy: a pseudogestational sac is seen in 10–20% of

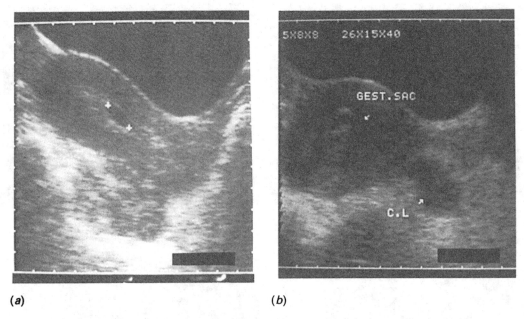

(a)   *(b)*

Figure 4.3 (*a*) Transabdominal ultrasound: longitudinal section of uterus
containing a small intrauterine gestation sac with asymmetrical trophoblast ring
(normal intrauterine pregnancy). (*b*) Transabdominal ultrasound: transverse section
of uterus containing an eccentrically located normal intrauterine gestation sac and
right-sided corpus luteum.

these cases (Figure 4.2a–c). This may reflect the hyperplastic endometrium of a pregnancy or may be a collection of blood within the uterine
cavity which lies in the centre of the cavity; it can thus be distinguished
from an early (pre-six weeks) intrauterine gestation sac, which is always
eccentric (Figure 4.3a,b). Arguments persist as to whether a pseudogestational sac is seen using TVS. In the experience of some (Timor-Tritsch *et
al.*, 1988), no pseudogestational sac is present in the uterus at the time at
which the early tubal gestation is detected. Others admit that it may be
difficult, even with TVS, to evaluate a very early intrauterine sac (less
than 4 mm in diameter). Eccentric placement within the endometrial
cavity is a hallmark of intrauterine nidation. In the absence of this,
especially if the uterine texture is homogeneous, a pseudogestational sac
should be suspected (Cacciatore *et al.*, 1989).

Characteristically, the eccentrically located early gestational sac is
surrounded by an asymmetrical trophoblast ring. This asymmetry
distinguishes normal pregnancy from an ectopic gestation and from
hormone-induced changes associated with the normal menstrual cycle.
The normal early intrauterine pregnancy may have a double sac

Box 4.2. Ultrasound features of failed intrauterine pregnancy.

1. Complete abortion: empty uterus
2. Incomplete abortion: collapsed gestation sac or thick irregular echoes in midline of uterine cavity
3. Anembryonic pregnancy: absence of embryonic echoes within a gestation sac large enough for such structures to be visible (mean sac diameter > 15 mm with TVS and 17 mm with TAS)
4. Early embryonic demise (missed abortion): absent heart action in embryo greater than 5 mm (TVS)

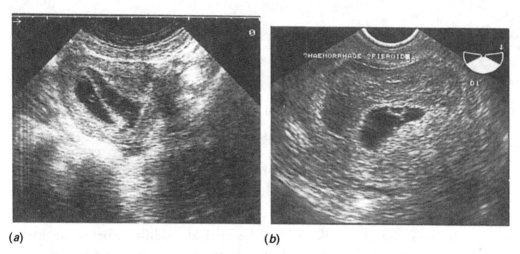

(*a*)   (*b*)

Figure 4.4 (*a*) and (*b*). Transvaginal ultrasound in threatened miscarriage: transverse section of uterus depicting a five-week gestation sac containing a yolk sac. There is a small intrauterine haemorrhage at the implantation site.

appearance because of the concentric decidua capsularis and parietalis (Bradley *et al.*, 1982). This feature may also be seen in one-third of ectopic pregnancies, thus limiting its usefulness in clinical practice (Nyberg *et al.*, 1988). The sonographic features of the various categories of failed intrauterine pregnancy are listed in Box 4.2.

Identification of the yolk sac may help to confirm the presence of an intrauterine pregnancy before a living embryo is detected (Figure 4.4). It is the first structure to be seen normally within the gestation sac appearing as a sphere a few millimeters in diameter. It is visible with TAS in all normal gestation sacs of mean diameter exceeding 20 mm (which corresponds to seven weeks amenorrhea). TVS allows earlier identification of the yolk sac, typically when the mean gestation sac diameter is greater than 8 mm (Levi *et al.*, 1988) or 10 mm (Cacciatore *et al.*, 1990).

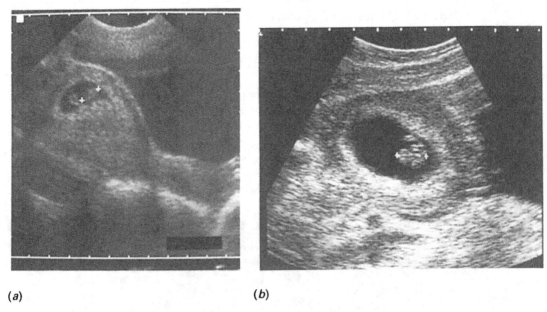

(a)   (b)

Figure 4.5 (*a*) Transabdominal ultrasound at 6.5 weeks' gestation.
(*b*) Transvaginal ultrasound depicting an intrauterine gestation sac containing a live embryo and yolk sac. Note that the yolk sac is located very close to the embryo and could easily be mistakenly added to the crown–rump measurement.

The presence of a yolk sac may be critical in differentiating an early intrauterine sac from a pseudosac (decidual cast), but its presence does not guarantee a normal pregnancy.

Careful inspection of the entire sac contents may be required to demonstrate the yolk sac, which is often found near the periphery of the sac. As the early embryo lies very close to the yolk sac at this stage of development, care should be taken to avoid including this structure in the measurement of crown–rump length (CRL), an error that could alter the measurement (and hence estimation of gestational age) by more than 50% (Figure 4.5).

It is possible to identify an embryo with a CRL as small as 1–3 mm using TVS (Figure 4.6). The corresponding figure for TAS is 5–6 mm, equivalent to six weeks gestation (Figure 4.7). Ultrasonographers have long reported the visualisation of cardiac activity using TAS even before the embryo is clearly identified. This is possible by careful examination of the yolk sac region (Cadkin and McAlpin, 1984). Using TVS, Bree et al. (1989) consistently demonstrated cardiac activity in all cases when pregnancy had advanced beyond 40 days from the LMP in patients with

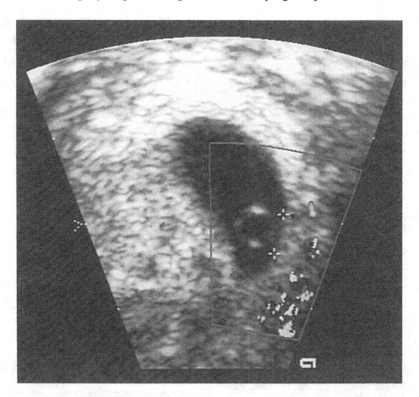

Figure 4.6 Transvaginal ultrasound of a five-week intrauterine pregnancy depicting a yolk sac. The patient had a 4 mm crown–rump length embryo (not seen).

reliable dates. In a longitudinal study basing ovulation on LH timing, TVS reliably detected an intrauterine sac by 33 days' gestation, a yolk sac by 38 days and embryonic echoes with a visible heart motion by 43 days (Cacciatore *et al.*, 1990). Reliable dates, however, are not a consistent feature in the obstetric population and detection of the LH surge is not as yet routine practice; one should therefore consider the smallest embryo size at which cardiac activity can consistently and reliably be determined. Using a 15 MHz TVS transducer in 363 normal singleton pregnancies, the earliest recorded cardiac activity (threshold value) occurred at 46 days from the LMP, at a mean sac diameter of 18.3 mm, an hCG level greater than 47 171 (First IRP) and a CRL of 3 mm (Rempen, 1990). It is easy to miss such early embryos: they appear as echogenic structures adjacent to the yolk sac at the periphery of the gestation sac. Embryos smaller than 5 mm may have visible cardiac activity, one-third of normal embryos with a CRL of less than 5 mm may not (Levi *et al.*, 1990; Pennell *et al.*, 1991).

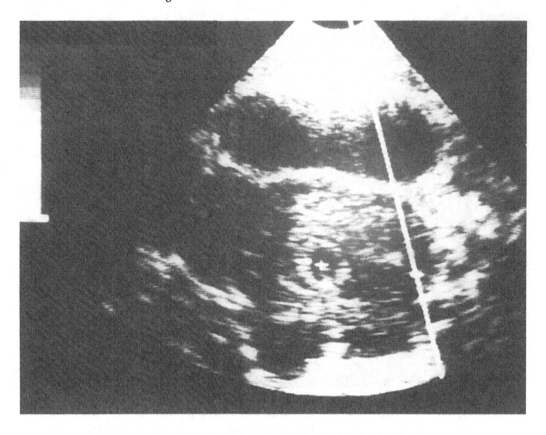

Figure 4.7 Transabdominal ultrasound of a six-week intrauterine pregnancy depicting a 6 mm crown–rump length embryo.

4.4   Sonographic features of ectopic pregnancy

4.4.1   TRANSABDOMINAL ULTRASOUND

The commonest use of ultrasound is to exclude ectopic pregnancy by visualisation of an intrauterine pregnancy. Although uncommon, imaging of the ectopic embryo with or without cardiac activity remains the gold standard for the sonographic diagnosis of ectopic pregnancy. Apart from live ectopic gestation (Figure 4.8), the diagnosis of ectopic pregnancy using abdominal ultrasound is fraught with difficulties (Stabile and Grudzinskas, 1990). Ectopic pregnancy may be suspected if there is an enlarged but empty uterus and/or an adnexal mass and/or fluid in the pouch of Douglas (Figure 4.9). Only rarely is it possible to distinguish between the causes of these abnormalities, such as inflammatory masses, cyst accidents and endometriosis, all of which may mimic an ectopic

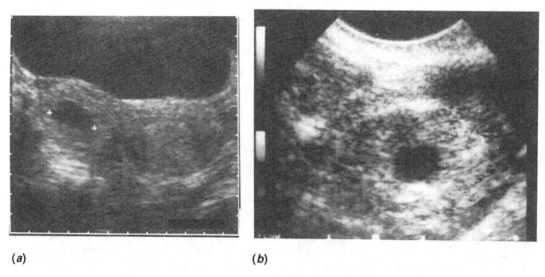

(*a*)   (*b*)

Figure 4.8 Transabdominal (*a*) and transvaginal (*b*) ultrasound of an ectopic pregnancy at seven weeks' gestation. The uterus contains thickened endometrium and the left adnexa contains an intact ring which represents the ectopic gestation. This pregnancy was anembryonic.

pregnancy. Minor pelvic abnormalities such as a simple ovarian cyst or small quantities of fluid in the pouch of Douglas are of no greater significance in the ultrasound diagnosis of ectopic pregnancy than no abnormality at all. The management of a pregnant woman with a non-diagnostic scan is described in Chapter 6.

We have previously reported that without knowing whether the patient is pregnant or not, in cases of suspected ectopic pregnancy, TAS provides an accurate diagnosis in 62% of ectopic pregnancies, with a specificity of 57% and a positive predictive value of 25%. In the absence of any ultrasound abnormality, there is an 87% probability of excluding this life-threatening condition (Stabile *et al.*, 1988). Similar results have been reported by others (Levi and Lebliq, 1980). Hence, even high resolution TAS cannot be recommended as the sole diagnostic test in a suspected ectopic pregnancy.

The issue of whether the combination of ultrasound with biochemical tests provides additional information of clinical importance than the two techniques used in isolation has been addressed using the principles of Bayesian analysis in Section 3.4. In summary, although the combination of TAS and hCG improves the predictive accuracy for ectopic pregnancy, the diagnosis is always easier with increasing gestational age and with the occurrence of rupture. Most studies that have addressed this issue fail to

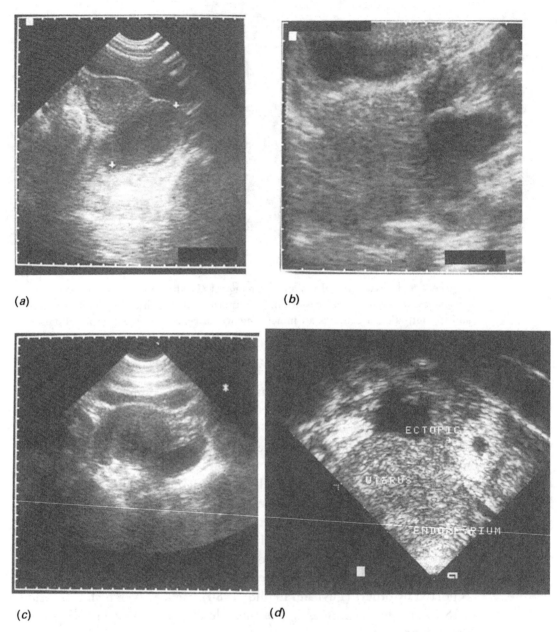

Figure 4.9 shows adnexal masses. (*a*) Transabdominal ultrasound: transverse section of uterus and right-sided simple adnexal mass. The patient had a corpus luetum cyst at laparoscopy. (*b*) Transabdominal ultrasound: transverse section of uterus and right-sided complex adnexal mass. The patient had a hydrosalpinx at laparoscopy. (*c*) Transabdominal ultrasound: transverse section of uterus and right-sided complex adnexal mass. The patient had an ectopic pregnancy at laparoscopy. (*d*) Transvaginal ultrasound: transverse section of uterus showing right ectopic pregnancy.

> **Box 4.3. Ultrasound features of ectopic pregnancy.**
>
> 1. Transabdominal ultrasound
>   - Live embryo in adnexa (10–12%)
>   - Pseudogestational sac in uterus
>   - Empty uterus +/− adnexal sac +/− fluid in pouch of Douglas
> 2. Transvaginal ultrasound
>   - Live ectopic: intact tubal ring with heart action (20%)
>   - Tubal abortion: poorly defined tubal ring +/− fluid in pouch of Douglas
>   - Ruptured tube: fluid in pouch of Douglas

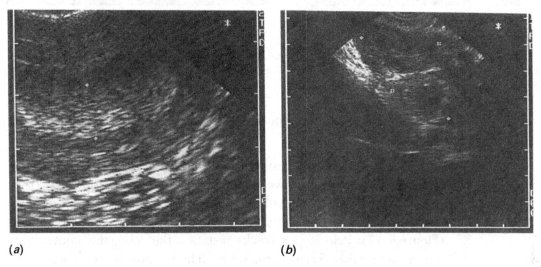

(a)   (b)

Figure 4.10 (*a*) Transvaginal ultrasound showing a coronal section of the uterus with a thickened endometrium. (*b*) Transvaginal ultrasound showing a parasagittal section of the right adnexa in the same patient. The intact tubal ring of an ectopic pregnancy is clearly visible.

point out that by the time TAS achieves good diagnostic accuracy, at least half the cases will have been diagnosed already and treated.

4.4.2   TRANSVAGINAL ULTRASOUND

Several excellent books describing the technique of TVS are available (Timor-Tritsch and Rottem, 1987; Kurjak, 1991; Fleischer and Kepple, 1992; Chervenak *et al.*, 1993), to which the interested reader is encouraged to refer.

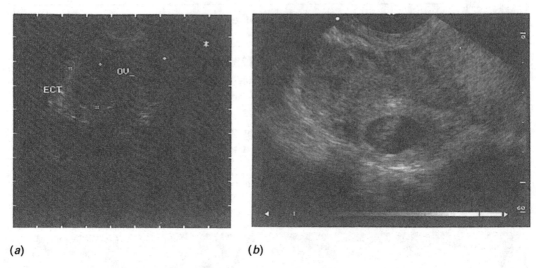

(a)   (b)

Figure 4.11 Transvaginal ultrasound showing an intact tubal ring (*a*) of an ectopic pregnancy with an embryo (*b*) at the upper pole.

There are three vaginosonographic features of tubal pregnancy (Box 4.3):

1. A live embryo within a gestational sac in the adnexa. This typically appears as an intact and well-defined tubal ring (Figure 4.10) (the 'bagel' sign) in which the yolk sac and/or the embryonic pole with or without cardiac action are seen within a completely sonolucent sac (Figure 4.11). Prior to six weeks gestation the echogenic contour of the sac is less than 5 mm in diameter. These features are identical to those seen via the abdominal route. In our prospective study of abdominal scanning, the diagnosis was made in 12% of patients with ectopic pregnancy, but only after seven weeks amenorrhea (Stabile *et al.*, 1988). The major advantage of TVS is said to be the earlier gestational age at which this diagnosis can be made; however many ectopic pregnancies may be anembryonic (Emmrich and Kopping, 1981), in which case TVS would not diagnose more intact viable ectopics than hitherto demonstrated.

2. A poorly-defined tubal ring (Figure 4.12) which sometimes contains echogenic structures ('complex adnexal mass'). The pouch of Douglas may contain fluid and/or blood. These are features of a tubal pregnancy that is aborting. A thickened tube containing a blood clot is often seen at surgery.

3. Varying amounts of fluid in the pouch of Douglas probably representing a ruptured tubal pregnancy. Echogenic fluid alone may be seen in

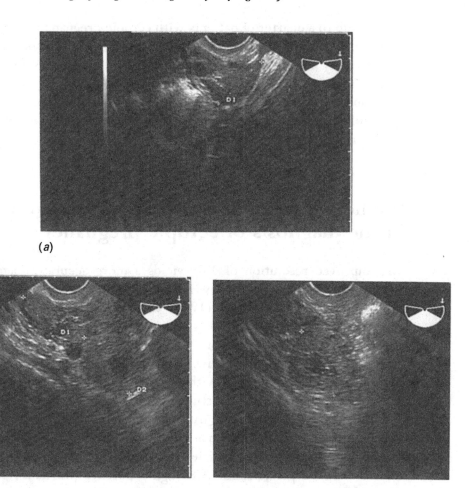

(a)

(b)   *(c)*

Figure 4.12 Transvaginal ultrasound of an ectopic pregnancy which is aborting.
A thickened tube containing blood clot was seen at laparotomy. (*a*) Left ovary.
(*b*) Right ovary. (*c*) Poorly defined tubal ring.

15% of patients with ectopic pregnancy (Nyberg *et al.*, 1991). The
tubal ring may not be seen, or may be blurred and unrecognisable
within the blood clot. Patients who have undergone ovulation
induction often have varying amounts of ascites which may be falsely
reported as blood.

One of the notable advantages of TVS is that it can be used as an
extension of the examining fingers as part of a bimanual examination.
Pelvic structures may be approximated to the tip of the probe using
the free hand and the probe can be used with care to locate the point of
maximum intensity of pain.

In up to a quarter of patients with ectopic pregnancy, TVS may be normal (Russell *et al.*, 1993). Short-term follow-up (one to seven days) may help as a small ectopic pregnancy may grow sufficiently to be visualised on a second scan. Although uncommon, the possibility of a non-tubal (cornual, interstitial or cervical) ectopic pregnancy should be considered, when none of the classical sonographic features described above is identified.

4.5   Predictive value of transvaginal sonography in the diagnosis of ectopic pregnancy

The improved resolution of TVS yields a more accurate diagnosis of intrauterine pregnancy with low false positive and false negative rates. The studies of DeCrespigny (1988) and Nyberg *et al.* (1991) have addressed the value of specific TVS abnormalities in women with clinically suspected ectopic pregnancy using transducers of identical frequency. The positive predictive value for ultrasonic parameters such as adnexal abnormalities with or without pelvic fluid were good (63–100%) in both studies; however in the study by DeCrespigny (1988), seven of 36 (19%) women with ectopic pregnancy had no detectable abnormalities on TVS. Similarly, 13 of 68 (19%) patients studied by Nyberg and colleagues had no extrauterine abnormalities such as an ectopic embryo, sac or adnexal mass or pelvic fluid. Although a positive pregnancy test was essential for entry into Nyberg's study, it did not improve the diagnostic value of TVS.

Russell and colleagues (1993) retrospectively studied 123 women clinically at risk for ectopic pregnancy (any combination of pain, bleeding or palpable mass with a positive pregnancy test), in an attempt to evaluate the impact of TVS on their practice. Nineteen women (15%) had a surgically proven ectopic pregnancy of which only three were directly visualised by TVS (2.4% of the study group). A quarter of the ectopics had a normal TVS at presentation and none of them had an adnexal ring. The combination of a pelvic mass and free fluid carried the highest risk for an ectopic pregnancy in this cohort (77%). In patients with a normal adnexa and no fluid in the pouch of Douglas, the risk for ectopic pregnancy was 33%, i.e. if the scan were normal, there was still a one in three risk that the patient had an ectopic pregnancy. An intrauterine pregnancy was correctly diagnosed in 74% of women at the initial scan, in comparison with 58% at the first TAS in an earlier study from the same unit (Mahoney *et al.*, 1985). The major benefit of TVS in this study was that a normal intrauterine pregnancy was recognised up to a week earlier; in many cases it did not permit a confident diagnosis of ectopic pregnancy.

In summary, TVS gives better image quality and improved detection of non-specific pelvic abnormalities, such as free fluid in the pouch of Douglas, adnexal masses etc. This is not necessarily, however, reflected in a better predictive value for ectopic pregnancy. For example, Bateman *et al.* (1990) have shown that the predictive value of an adnexal mass for ectopic pregnancy may be lower when detectable by TVS than TAS. Thus the test may improve the sensitivity for ectopic pregnancy, but the specificity may be lower. This disadvantage may be offset by the value of TVS in reducing the number of non-diagnostic scans in women with positive pregnancy tests. TVS undoubtedly reduces the necessity for repeat testing.

4.6　Transvaginal sonography, transabdominal sonography or both?

Patients with ruptured tubal pregnancy (Group 1) are often in shock and require urgent resuscitation before emergency surgery. Abdominal ultrasound is not practical in this situation, partly because of the delay in filling the bladder and poor image quality, especially in the obese patient. Using TVS, by contrast, it takes only a few seconds to recognise the unmistakable appearance of a blood clot in the pelvis. Patients with subacute ectopic pregnancy presenting with non-specific symptoms and signs (Group 3) typically have a complex adnexal mass on ultrasound, although a viable ectopic pregnancy in the adnexa is found in approximately 20% of cases (DeCrespigny, 1988).

Given the limitations described in Section 4.1, the consensus view is that ectopic pregnancy is more frequently identified using TVS than TAS (Shapiro *et al.*, 1988), and that intrauterine pregnancy is diagnosed at an earlier stage. Thus surgery may be avoided in pregnant patients with a haemorrhagic cyst of the corpus luteum (Figure 4.13). Complex adnexal masses may be seen in 7% of patients with a normal intrauterine pregnancy (Nyberg *et al.*, 1991). If large adnexal cysts extend above the bladder into the lower abdomen, the transvaginal technique may be at a disadvantage. In addition, when abdominal pregnancy is suspected, abdominal scanning is preferable unless the gestational sac implants in the pelvis. This is exceedingly rare (Chapter 7).

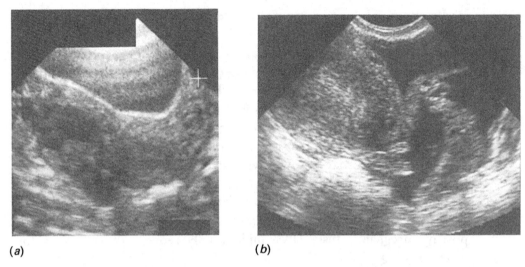

(a)   (b)

Figure 4.13 Transabdominal ultrasound (a) showing transverse section of uterus and left-sided haemorrhagic corpus luteum cyst. This is less likely to be confused with an ectopic pregnancy if the patient is scanned vaginally (b).

With the earlier diagnosis of ectopic pregnancy, fewer of them will have ruptured at the time of presentation and surgery can be more conservative. It has yet to be demonstrated, however, that widespread use of TVS (i.e. not just in the hands of experts in tertiary centres) leads to a reduction in the morbidity and mortality of this life-threatening condition. Indeed, even in the best of hands (DeCrespigny, 1988; Shapiro *et al.*, 1988; Cacciatore *et al.*, 1989; Nyberg *et al.*, 1991; Russell *et al.*, 1993), up to a quarter of women have no vaginosonographic abnormalities (false negatives). This figure may fall as experience with TVS increases.

4.7   Limitations of transvaginal sonography

Most patients, especially those used to the discomforts of a full bladder, find that TVS is no more uncomfortable than a speculum examination. In some countries, patient education and custom may limit its acceptability. Other disadvantages of TVS include the small field of view and the limited mobility of the probe. In up to 50% of patients, direct TVS visualisation of an ectopic pregnancy may be difficult or confusing, such that the abnormality may be incompletely seen or missed altogether, particularly by an inexperienced operator (Parvey and Maklad, 1993).

Common pitfalls include the following. 1. The intact tubal ring may be confused with the corpus luteum of pregnancy, a graafian follicle, loops of

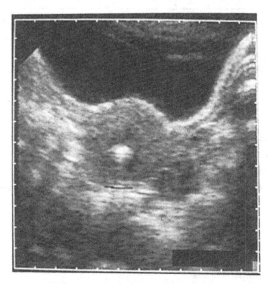

Figure 4.14 Transabdominal ultrasound showing transverse section of uterus containing an intrauterine contraceptive device which masked the ectopic pregnancy.

small bowel or other tubal pathology such as a hydrosalpinx imaged in cross-section. These mistakes are made most often when a static film is interpreted. Most can be eliminated by inspection of real time images. The corpus luteum and graafian follicle can be identified by defining the ovary itself. Peristalsis can be seen in the small bowel, helping to avoid this mistake. 2. Unless the myometrium of the uterus is identified (which can be surprisingly difficult on occasions), the beginner may miss the tubal gestation altogether. 3. All or part of the tube may be invisible acoustically if there is no fluid to outline the pelvic viscera. 4. Camouflage by adjacent structures may occur when an adnexal ectopic pregnancy is largely solid. Asymmetrical enlargement of one ovary may be the only clue. These and other errors can be minimised by meticulous examination of multiple and reproducible sections.

Apart from the significant false negative rate of TVS, Goldstein *et al.* (1988) identified a subgroup of patients which was difficult to evaluate. An unselected group of 235 potentially normal early pregnancies presenting to an abortion clinic included 10 pregnant women (hCG levels between 394 and 6000 IU/L), in whom TVS failed to demonstrate an intrauterine sac. Two of these women had an ectopic pregnancy, although in one the diagnosis was sonographically obvious due to an extrauterine sac. There were also three missed abortions (early embryonic demise), two complete abortions and three normal intrauterine pregnancies in the group. All three normal pregnancies missed by TVS were associated with

---

Box 4.4. Interpretation of hCG results in suspected ectopic pregnancy (EP).

hCG negative: EP excluded if sensitive assay is used

hCG positive: proceed to TVS

1. Normal intrauterine pregnancy; exclude heterotopic pregnancy
2. Empty gestational sac (mean sac diameter < 1.5 cm):
   - (a) Failed intrauterine pregnancy (anembryonic pregnancy): repeat U/S in one week to confirm
   - (b) Pregnancy too early to visualise yolk sac ($<$ day 38), embryonic pole with embryonic heat action (< 43 days): repeat U/S
3. Normal pelvis:
   - (a) False positive hCG: repeat test
   - (b) Normal or ectopic pregnancy too early to visualise: serial quantitative hCG estimations
4. Complex adnexal mass $+/-$ free fluid in pouch of Douglas: probable EP

---

either a fibroid uterus or a co-existing intrauterine device, which presumably masked the intrauterine sac (Figure 4.14). These results also emphasise that when the uterus appears empty at an hCG level above the accepted discriminatory zone for TVS, then ultrasound cannot distinguish between the various types of pregnancy failure (Box 4.4).

4.8   Conclusion

Ultrasound examinations are highly operator dependent. TVS can provide virtually instantaneous answers to some, but not all, difficult clinical problems. After adequate training TVS is simple, acceptable and provides improved resolution. At least in the hands of experts in tertiary centres (most likely to publish their results) it leads to earlier diagnosis of ectopic pregnancy in at least 50% of cases. It remains to be seen whether this is also true of ultrasound departments in all units. In addition TVS does not require a full bladder: in an emergency the patient can be kept fasted and surgery is not delayed. The possibility of a non-tubal (cornual, interstitial or cervical) ectopic pregnancy should be considered when none of the classical sonographic features is identified. When abdominal pregnancy is suspected, abdominal scanning is preferable unless the gestational sac implants in the pelvis.

4.9   **Point summary**

1. Ultrasound is used to locate the site of pregnancy in women with a positive hCG.

2. Normal intrauterine pregnancy virtually excludes the diagnosis of ectopic pregnancy, although a combination occurs once in every 4000–7000 pregnancies.

3. Direct sonographic diagnosis of ectopic pregnancy is only possible in 20% of cases, even with TVS. In a further 20–25% of cases there may be no ultrasound abnormalities.

4. A normal intrauterine pregnancy can be seen up to a week earlier by TVS than with TAS.

5. TVS reduces the number of non-diagnostic or unhelpful scans in women with positive pregnancy tests.

6. Failed intrauterine pregnancy may be indistinguishable from ectopic pregnancy using either TAS or TVS.

7. Negative or normal TVS examination does not exclude the presence of ectopic pregnancy.

8. Interpretation of the test result should take into account the method of conception and the mode of clinical presentation.

9. No single method/test available today is able to correctly diagnose or exclude ectopic pregnancy every time it is suspected.

4.10   **References**

Andolf, E., Jorgensen, C. (1990). A prospective comparison of transabdominal and transvaginal ultrasound with surgical findings in gynecological disease. *Journal of Ultrasound in Medicine*, **9**: 71–75.

Bateman, B.G., Nunley, W.C., Kolp, L.A. (1990). Vaginal sonography and hCG dynamics of early intrauterine and tubal pregnancies. *Obstetrics and Gynecology*, **75**: 421–427.

Bernaschek, G., Rudelstorfer, R., Csaicsich, P. (1988). Vaginal sonography versus serum hCG in early detection of pregnancy. *American Journal of Obstetrics and Gynecology*, **158**: 608–612.

Bradley, W.G., Fiske, C.E., Filly, R.A. (1982). The double sac sign of early intrauterine pregnancy: use in exclusion of ectopic pregnancy. *Radiology*, **143**: 223–226.

Bree, L.R., Edwards, M., Bohm Velez, M., Beyler, S., Roberts, J., Mendelson, A. B. (1989). Transvaginal sonography in the evaluation of normal early pregnancy: correlation with hCG level. *American Journal of Radiology*, **153**: 75–79.

Cacciatore, B., Tiitinen, A., Stenman, D.H., Ylostalo, P. (1990). Normal early pregnancy: serum hCG levels and vaginal ultrasonography findings. *British Journal of Obstetrics and Gynecology*, **97**: 899–903.

Cacciatore, B., Stenman, U-H., Ylostalo, P. (1989). Comparison of abdominal and vaginal sonography in suspected ectopic pregnancy. *Obstetrics and Gynecology*, **73**: 770–774.

Cadkin, A.V., McAlpin, R.T. (1984). Detection of fetal cardiac activity between 41 and 43 days of gestation. *Journal of Ultrasound in Medicine*, **3**: 499–503.

Chervenak, F., Isaacson, G.C., Campbell, S. (1993). *Ultrasound in Obstetrics and Gynecology*. Little Brown and Company, Boston.

Coleman, B.G., Arger, P.H., Grumbach, K. (1988). Transvaginal and transabdominal sonography: prospective comparison. *Radiology*, **166**: 639–644.

DeCrespigny, L. (1988). Early diagnosis of pregnancy failure with transvaginal ultrasound. *American Journal of Obstetrics and Gynecology*, **159**: 408–409.

Emmrich, P., Kopping, H. (1981). A study of placental villi in extrauterine gestation: a guide to the frequency of blighted ova. *Placenta*, **2**: 63–70.

Fleischer, A.C., Kepple, D.M. (1992). *Transvaginal Sonography. A Clinical Atlas*. J B Lippincott, Philadelphia.

Goldstein, S.R., Snyder, J.R., Watson, C., Danon, M. (1988). Very early pregnancy detection with endovaginal ultrasound. *Obstetrics and Gynecology*, **72**: 200–204.

Jain, K.A., Hamper, U.M., Sanders, R.C. (1988). Comparison of transvaginal and transabdominal sonography in the detection of an early pregnancy and its complications. *American Journal of Radiology*, **151**: 1139–1143.

Kurjak, A. (1991). *Transvaginal Color Doppler*. The Parthenon Publishing Group, New Jersey.

Lande, I.M., Hill, M.C., Cosco, E.E. (1988). Adnexal and cul-de-sac abnormalities: transvaginal sonography. *Radiology*, **166**: 325–332.

Levi, C.S., Lebliq, P. (1980). The diagnostic value of ultrasonography in 342 cases of suspected ectopic pregnancy. *Acta Obstetrica Gynaecologica Scandinava*, **59**: 29–31.

Levi, C.S., Lyons, E.A., Lindsay, D.J. (1988). Early diagnosis of non-viable pregnancy with endovaginal ultrasound. *Radiology*, **167**: 383–385.

Levi, C.S., Lyons, E.A., Zheng, X.H., Lindsay, D.J., Holt, S.C. (1990). Endovaginal ultrasound demonstration of cardiac activity in embryos of less than 5 mm in crown rump length. *Radiology*, **176**: 71–74.

Liebman, J.A., Kruse, B., McSweeney, M.B (1988). Transvaginal sonography: comparison with transabdominal sonography in the diagnosis of pelvic masses. *American Journal of Radiology*, **151**: 89–92.

Mahoney, B.S., Filly, R.A., Nyberg, D.A (1985). Sonographic evaluation of ectopic pregnancy. *Journal of Ultrasound in Medicine*, **4**: 221–228.

Mendelson, E.B., Bohm-Velez, M., Joseph, N. (1988). Gynecologic imaging: comparison of transabdominal and transvaginal sonography. *Radiology*, **166**: 321–324.

Nyberg, D.A., Hughes, M.P., Mack, L., Wang, K.W. (1991). Extrauterine findings of ectopic pregnancy at transvaginal ultrasound: importance of echogenic fluid. *Radiology*, **178**: 823–826.

Nyberg, D.A., Mack, L.A., Laing, F.C., Jeffrey, R.B (1988). Early pregnancy complications: endovaginal sonographic findings correlated with human chorionic gonadotropin levels. *Radiology*, **167**: 619–622.

Parvey, H.R., Maklad, N. (1993). Pitfalls in the transvaginal sonographic diagnosis of ectopic pregnancy. *Journal of Ultrasound in Medicine*, **12**: 139–144.

Pennell, R.C., Baltarowich, O.H., Kurtz, A.B., Vilaro, M.M. (1987). Complicated first trimester pregnancies: evaluation with endovaginal versus transabdominal technique. *Radiology*, **165**: 79–83.

Pennell, R.C., Needleman, L., Pajak, T., Baltarowich, O., Vilaro, M., Goldberg, B.B., Kurtz, A.B. (1991). Prospective comparison of vaginal and abdominal sonography in normal early pregnancy. *Journal of Ultrasound in Medicine*, **10**(2): 63–67.

Rempen, A. (1988). Vaginal sonography in ectopic pregnancy: a prospective evaluation. *Journal of Ultrasound in Medicine*, **7**: 381–387.

Rempen, A. (1990). Diagnosis of viability in early pregnancy with vaginal sonography. *Journal of Ultrasound in Medicine*, **9**(12): 711–716.

Russell, S.A., Filly, R.A., Damato, N. (1993). Sonographic diagnosis of ectopic pregnancy with endovaginal probes: what really has changed? *Journal of Ultrasound in Medicine*, **3**: 145–153.

Shapiro, B.B., Cullen, M., Taylor, K.J.W., deCherney, A.H. (1988). Transvaginal ultrasound for the diagnosis of ectopic pregnancy. *Fertility and Sterility*, **50**: 425–429.

Stabile, I. (1992). Diagnosis and management of ectopic pregnancy. In: *Spontaneous Abortion: Diagnosis and Treatment*, (ed I. Stabile, J.G. Grudzinskas, T. Chard), pp. 159–182. Springer-Verlag, London.

Stabile, I., Campbell, S., Grudzinskas, J.G. (1988). Can ultrasound reliably diagnose ectopic pregnancy? *British Journal of Obstetrics and Gynaecology*,

95: 1247–1252.

Stabile, I., Grudzinskas, J.G. (1990). Ectopic pregnancy: a review of incidence, etiology and diagnostic aspects. *Obstetrics and Gynecology Survey*, **45**(6): 335–347.

Timor-Tritsch, I.E., Rottem, S. (1987). *Transvaginal Sonography*. Elsevier, New York.

Timor-Tritsch, I.E., Rottem, S., Thaler, I. (1988). Review of transvaginal sonography: a description with clinical application. *Ultrasound Quarterly*, **8**: 1–34.

Yeh, H.C., Goodman, J.D., Carr, L., Rabinowitz, J.G. (1986). Intradecidual sign: an ultrasound criterion of early intrauterine pregnancy. *Radiology*, **161**: 463–467.

CHAPTER 5

Surgical diagnosis

In resume, to diagnose a suspected or unruptured ectopic pregnancy, the history should be properly evaluated and a certain sequence of procedures followed. A biological test for pregnancy should be made, followed by pelvic examination under anesthesia. In the presence of a definite adnexal mass, no evidence of a blighted ovum on curettage and a positive test for pregnancy, a laparotomy may be performed forthwith. Otherwise, if there is still doubt, culdoscopy or surgical exploration of the posterior cul-de-sac should be performed, with subsequent treatment depending upon the findings.

J.B. de Lee, 1933

5.1   Introduction

This chapter will describe other methods available for the diagnosis of ectopic pregnancy. In the western world, most of these methods have now been superseded by non-invasive biochemical and sonographic modalities.

5.2   Culdocentesis

Culdocentesis, whether pre- or intraoperatively, was widely used, particularly in the USA, to detect blood in the pouch of Douglas. With the patient in the lithotomy position, an 18 gauge needle is inserted through the posterior fornix and any blood/fluid present is aspirated. The test is rapid but painful. The test is positive if non-clotting blood with a haematocrit of more than 10% is obtained, negative if clear or blood-tinged fluid and non-diagnostic if no blood or fluid is obtained. In one study, 80% of patients with an ectopic pregnancy had a positive test, 2% had a negative result and in 16% the test was non-diagnostic (Romero et al., 1985). Clearly, before the advent of ultrasonography, there were few other clues as to whether mild to minimal intraperitoneal bleeding (found in up to 80–95% of proven ectopic pregnancies, both ruptured and unruptured) had occurred, hence the rationale behind this procedure. Non-clotting blood reflects active bleeding, which may come from an ectopic pregnancy, a ruptured ovarian cyst and even retrograde menstruation (up to 300 ml of menstrual blood may be found in the pouch of Douglas; POD) or endometriosis. The false positive rate of this procedure ranges from 5% to 10%. Attempts to reduce this by repeating the procedure or by other diagnostic tests such as culdoscopy (Breen, 1970) or colpotomy (Draa and Baum, 1951) are now obsolete. Only half of the patients with positive culdocentesis presented with evidence of peritoneal irritation (Romero *et al.*, 1985). Of greater concern is the false negative rate of 11–14%. This arises because unless the procedure is performed in the reverse Trendelenburg position, blood may not be obtained at culdocentesis even if a haemoperitoneum is present. Intact unruptured ectopic pregnancies account for the remaining false negatives. Ultrasound and laparoscopy have made this procedure obsolete.

5.3   Dilatation and Curettage

Dilatation and curettage is the most frequently performed operation in gynaecology. Pelvic examination precedes insertion of the uterine sound. After careful dilatation to 7–10 mm, the uterine cavity is explored and systematically curetted. Complications include: (1) laceration of the cervix; (2) primary or secondary haemorrhage; (3) perforation of the uterus with or without peritonitis, peritonism, bowel damage or haemorrhage into the broad ligament; (4) pelvic cellulitis and parametritis; and (5) Asherman's syndrome (intrauterine adhesions).

In the past, when ectopic pregnancy was suspected, traditional surgical teaching included curetting the uterus to determine whether villi were present prior to laparotomy. The presence of chorionic villi indicated intrauterine pregnancy, whether ongoing or failed. In addition, the finding of decidua without chorionic villi in the uterus was considered strong presumptive evidence of an ectopic pregnancy. A generous amount of endometrium showing complete decidual change might be expected in an ectopic pregnancy, although this is rarely found, either because the patient has bled prior to presentation or because the the syncytium is not viable. A scanty endometrium or lack of decidual reaction, therefore, does not exclude the diagnosis of ectopic pregnancy. High false positive and false negative rates are associated with this 'diagnostic' test. There is also a good reason to avoid curetting the uterus in cases of a very early suspected ectopic pregnancy. If the pelvis was examined by means of

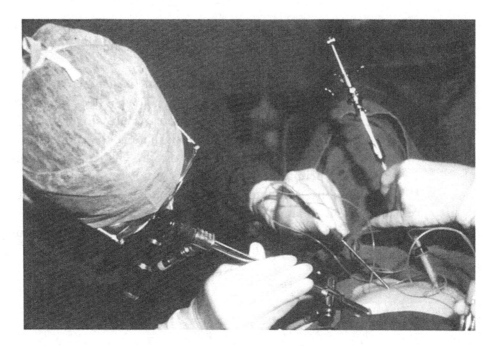

Figure 5.1 Laparoscopy: the gynaecologist employs a three-puncture technique to examine the pelvis using a laparoscope (right-hand) while mobilising other organs with the left hand. An assistant helps.

abdominal ultrasound, an early intrauterine pregnancy may have been missed. In this case, if the laparoscopy fails to detect an ectopic pregnancy, the intrauterine manipulation may disturb the early intrauterine pregnancy. There is no place for routine use of this procedure in modern clinical practice.

5.4   Laparoscopy

Laparoscopy may be used diagnostically and/or therapeutically. A pneumoperitoneum is produced by insufflating 2–4 L of carbon dioxide through a Veress needle inserted subumbilically. The laparoscope is inserted via the trochar. Other instruments are inserted into the abdominal cavity to improve organ handling and to perform endoscopic surgery such as haemostasis, adhesiolysis, linear salpingostomy, etc. (Figure 5.1). The procedure is typically performed without an intrauterine manipulator, so as to avoid disturbing a possible co-existing intrauterine pregnancy. Both tubes must be visualised in their entirety to avoid missing the pregnancy. If adhesions impair the view, laparotomy should follow as half these patients have an ectopic pregnancy (Esposito, 1980). Complications of laparoscopy include vascular, bowel and urinary tract injury.

Laparoscopy is considered the optimal invasive method to both diagnose and exclude an ectopic pregnancy, and has been shown to reduce the rate of ruptured ectopic pregnancies (Helvacioglu *et al.*, 1979). Laparoscopy provides a positive diagnosis in more than 90% of cases (Kim *et al.*, 1987) with a false positive rate of 5%. The diagnosis is missed in 3–4% of cases, primarily in very early ectopic pregnancies (Yaffe *et al.*, 1979). Adhesions, extreme obesity and poor technique account for the remaining cases. If an ectopic pregnancy is not found at laparoscopy, the procedure is often warranted anyway for the diagnosis of other surgically treatable conditions, e.g. haemosalpinx or torsion of an adnexal mass on its pedicle.

5.5   Point summary

1. Culdocentesis is positive if non-clotting blood with a haematocrit of more than 10% is obtained.

2. The false positive rate of culdocentesis is 5–10% and the false negative rate is 11–14%.

3. Laparoscopy reduces the rate of ruptured ectopic pregnancies. It has a false negative rate of 3–4% and false positive rate of 5%.

5.6   References

Breen, J. (1970). A 21-year survey of 654 ectopic pregnancies. *American Journal of Obstetrics and Gynecology*, **106**: 1004–1019.

Draa, C.C., Baum, H.C. (1951). Posterior colpotomy: an aid in the diagnosis and treatment of ectopic pregnancy. *American Journal of Obstetrics and Gynecology*, **61**: 300–311.

De Lee, J.B. (1933). *Principles and Practice of Obstetrics*. W.B. Saunders, Philadelphia.

Esposito, V.M. (1980). Ectopic pregnancy: the laparoscope as a diagnostic aid. *Journal of Reproductive Medicine*, **25**: 17–23.

Helvacioglu, A., Long, E.M., Yang, S-L. (1979). Ectopic pregnancy: an eight-year review. *Journal of Reproductive Medicine*, **22**: 87–92.

Kim, D.S., Chung, S.R., Park, M.I., Kim, Y.P. (1987). Comparative review of diagnostic accuracy in tubal pregnancy: a 14-year survey of 1040 cases. *Obstetrics and Gynecology*, **70**(4): 547–54.

Romero, R., Copel, J.A., Kadar, N. (1985). The value of culdocentesis in the diagnosis of ectopic pregnancy. *Obstetrics and Gynecology*, **65**: 519–522.

Yaffe, H., Navot, D., Laufer, N. (1979). Pitfalls in early detection of ectopic pregnancy. *Lancet*, **1**: 227–229.

CHAPTER 6

Practical management of suspected ectopic pregnancy

6.1 Introduction

The missed diagnosis of an ectopic pregnancy accounts for a significant proportion of all malpractice dollar losses in the USA, in part because of the high incidence of the condition and the serious consequences of missing the diagnosis. This high risk of professional liability has led to increasing pressure on gynaecologists to request more and more tests with little regard to resource implications. This chapter addresses the practical management of a suspected ectopic pregnancy in the litigious climate of the 1990s. We shall first examine the diagnostic strategies available in different clinical subgroups. This is followed by a section on the value of very early diagnosis of ectopic pregnancy (i.e. before six weeks of pregnancy).

6.2 Symptomatic but clinically stable women: combining ultrasound with biochemical tests

Pelvic sonography and a pregnancy test are often combined to evaluate early pregnancy complications. When attempting to locate the site of pregnancy in a woman with a positive test, attention must be paid to several points. The first is that assuming the human chorionic gonadotrophin (hCG) levels double every two days, there is a delay of 12–14 days between the biochemical detection of implantation (hCG more than 10 IU/L) and the identification of a gestational sac by transvaginal sonography (TVS) at hCG levels of more than 1000 IU/L (longer delay using transabdominal sonography; TAS). As a result of improvements in the technical quality of available ultrasound equipment, the threshold hCG level at which a gestational sac is always seen has fallen from

6500 IU/L (International Reference Preperation; IRP) with TAS to approximately 1000 IU/L (IRP) with TVS (Soussis *et al.*, 1991). Despite this marked improvement in ultrasound quality, there is a point at which it is not possible to identify an intrauterine gestation sac with the current state-of-the-art ultrasound equipment; definitive sonographic diagnosis will have to be delayed by a few days when the scan is repeated.

The second problem is that many patients at risk for ectopic pregnancy have an initial hCG value below the accepted discriminatory level. For example, 13% of patients suspected of harbouring an ectopic pregnancy initially presented with an hCG value of less than 1300 IU/L (IRP) (Stiller *et al.*, 1989); half of a group of patients with ectopic pregnancy had hCG levels of less than 750 IU/L (second IS) (DiMarchi *et al.*, 1989); and almost 70% had titres below 1500 IU/L (IRP) (Parvey and Maklad, 1993). It is expected that as the discriminatory hCG level falls, so will the proportion of patients in this category.

Using TVS, the intrauterine gestation sac is consistently seen when 2–4 mm in diameter, often only a week after the missed period, at which time the hCG level is approximately 1000 IU/L (IRP). Prior to that time the absence of a gestation sac neither increases nor decreases the possibility of an ectopic pregnancy. The intrauterine sac of a normal ongoing pregnancy should contain a yolk sac at 33 days, embryonic echoes at 38 days and visible heart activity at 43 days from the last menstrual period (LMP) (Cacciatore *et al.*, 1990b).

6.2.1   DIAGNOSTIC SCAN IN A PREGNANT WOMAN

Any woman with a positive pregnancy test and features suggestive of an ectopic pregnancy should have an ultrasound scan, provided the delay does not jeopardise her life (e.g. patients in Group 1). A number of possible scenarios follow. First, if the pregnancy is unequivocally located within the uterus (Figure 6.1), attention should turn to the adnexae to exclude a concomitant ectopic pregnancy, especially in women conceiving with the help of assisted reproductive techniques. Provided symptoms settle spontaneously, little else is necessary. The management of heterotopic pregnancy is discussed in Section 6.5.

Second, the scan may show an empty intrauterine gestation sac (Figure 6.2). This may represent a normal pregnancy at a stage too early to visualise its contents, or it may be a failed intrauterine pregnancy, e.g. spontaneous abortion in various stages of evolution, anembryonic sac or missed abortion (Stabile and Campbell, 1992). The sonographic features of these are listed in Box 4.3. It is essential to ensure that the sac is not

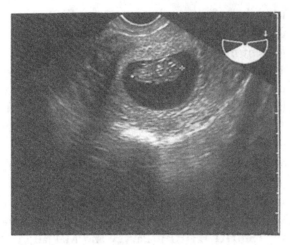

Figure 6.1 Ongoing intrauterine pregnancy.

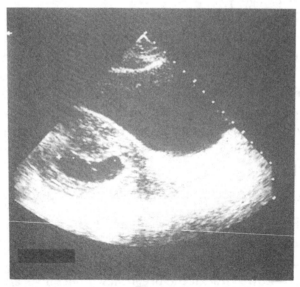

Figure 6.2 An empty intrauterine gestation sac.

pseudogestational. The diagnosis is obvious in most cases of failed intrauterine pregnancy that are examined by TVS but not by TAS. TVS should be performed if there is any doubt about the diagnosis. If the scan is unavailable or unhelpful (non-diagnostic) the patient should be managed as described in Section 6.2.2.

Third, the scan may show an apparently normal pelvis. This may be due to a false positive pregnancy test, in which case it should be repeated, or it may be too early to visualise the pregnancy, whether ectopic or

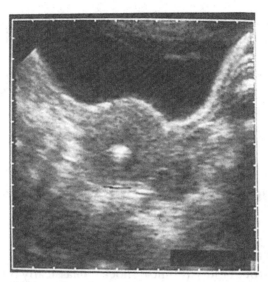

Figure 6.3 Transverse section of uterus containing an intrauterine contraceptive device and right-sided complex adnexal mass. The patient had a ectopic pregnancy at laparoscopy.

intrauterine. In patients in Group 2, intensive surveillance may be warranted. Clinical deterioration in patients at risk for an ectopic pregnancy would prompt many gynaecologists to carry out a laparoscopy.

Fourth, the scan may show a complex adnexal mass separate from the ovary with or without fluid in the pouch of Douglas (Figure 6.3). TVS may show that the adnexal mass contains a gestation sac, which is sometimes well defined and has an embryonic pole with or without cardiac activity, but more often is poorly defined and difficult to delineate. All these cases deserve laparoscopy.

The combination of an adnexal abnormality on ultrasound with a positive beta hCG has a sensitivity of 96%, specificity and positive predictive value of 100% and negative predictive value of 92% for ectopic pregnancy (Cacciatore *et al.*, 1990a, 1994; Fleisher *et al.*, 1990).

6.2.2   NON-DIAGNOSTIC SCAN IN A PREGNANT WOMAN

The management of this situation is identical whether using abdominal or vaginal ultrasound. If TAS and TVS are unhelpful, the next step is a quantitative hCG test. If the level is above the discriminatory zone appropriate to the type of ultrasound used, then laparoscopy is indicated. If the level is below the discriminatory zone, a repeat test should be performed not less than 48 hours later to determine the rate of increase. Interpretation of the results of serial hCG testing is described in Section

3.2.5. If quantitative hCG estimations are not available and the patient is in Group 3 (i.e., subacute symptoms only), then the scan should be repeated a few days later, preferably using TVS to determine whether the pregnancy is now visible. Should the clinical situation change in the interim, most gynaecologists would resort to laparoscopy. Curettage should be avoided especially if TAS rather than TVS were used to examine the pelvis.

6.3   Acute abdomen: emergency laparoscopy and laparotomy

Less than a quarter of patients with an ectopic pregnancy initially present with peripheral circulatory failure (clinical shock). Classically the patient is pale, grey and sometimes cyanotic. She lies still and has beads of sweat on her skin. The pupils are dilated and react slowly to light. Her temperature is below normal and her skin feels cool. Her pulse is rapid and thready and her blood pressure is lower than usual. Her superficial veins may be collapsed. Rapid intraperitoneal bleeding may irritate the peritoneum by collecting under the diaphragm causing shoulder tip pain; blood collecting in the pouch of Douglas may cause an urge to defaecate. Haemoperitoneum following rupture of the tube may be life-threatening. The differential diagnosis of internal bleeding includes ectopic pregnancy, ruptured spleen and a bleeding peptic ulcer. Haemorrhagic shock is the commonest reason for the high mortality rate associated with ectopic pregnancy (May *et al.*, 1976). In one study over half the women who died from ectopic pregnancy received no treatment and over 80% died of haemorrhage (Atrash *et al.*, 1987).

If available, detection of hCG points to an ectopic pregnancy as the cause of the internal bleeding. The emergency situation, however, dictates rapid transfer to the operating theatre for diagnostic laparoscopy or laparotomy. The increased awareness of ectopic pregnancy, earlier referral and the greater availability of diagnostic tests has resulted in this type of clinical presentation being now uncommon in the western world.

6.4   High risk group: intensive surveillance

Less than 20% of women with ectopic pregnancy are asymptomatic but at risk because of a past history of ectopic pregnancy (there is a recurrence rate of approximately 10%), previous tubal surgery or assisted conception; however, even if one or more of these risk factors is present, intrauterine pregnancy remains the likeliest diagnosis. Intensive surveillance (repeated hCG tests and TVS examinations) is warranted in this small group of women but reliance on high risk features alone is unlikely to pick up these cases (Section 6.6).

6.5   Suspected heterotopic pregnancy

Early diagnosis of a heterotopic pregnancy is only possible if a high degree of vigilance is maintained in all women who are at risk, primarily those conceiving after assisted conception. Heterotopic pregnancy also occurs in up to one in 4000 spontaneous conceptions (Hann *et al.*, 1984). Diagnosis is often delayed by attributing symptoms such as pain and bleeding to complications of the co-existent intrauterine pregnancy. As with ectopic pregnancy, the diagnosis will be missed unless it is considered in the differential diagnosis of abdominal pain in all women of reproductive age. Even if a gestation sac is seen in the uterus, the ultrasonographer should methodically examine the rest of the pelvis to exclude the possibility of a co-existing ectopic pregnancy. Biochemical tests such as hCG are not usually helpful, as levels are often in the normal range. Occasionally the diagnosis is only made at laparoscopy when careful examination reveals a pregnant uterus.

6.6   Very early diagnosis of ectopic pregnancy

The purpose of a very early diagnosis of ectopic pregnancy (i.e. before six weeks of pregnancy) is to prevent tubal damage and hence reduce the possibility of subsequent morbidity and allow conservative treatment aimed at preserving fertility. The first step in very early diagnosis is to identify those patients at risk (Box 1.2). Highly sensitive pregnancy tests can be used to demonstrate the presence or absence of a pregnancy-related disorder in virtually 100% of all cases (Seppala and Purhonen, 1987). If hCG is detected in either serum or urine, the next step is endovaginal ultrasound. Several studies, among which the elegant prospective study of Cacciatore *et al.* (1990b), have confirmed that vaginal sonography is associated with a sensitivity of 93% for ectopic pregnancy on admission, rising to 100% after repeat scanning. Even very small ectopic pregnancies, i.e. smaller than 1 cm in diameter were consistently visualised in this study, with a specificity of 99% and a 7% rate of ruptured ectopic pregnancy.

Symptomatic patients with a positive pregnancy test in whom no intrauterine pregnancy, adnexal mass or cul-de-sac fluid is detectable by TVS remain a diagnostic problem. A recent complete or incomplete miscarriage are possibilities as are an early viable intrauterine or ectopic pregnancy. In such cases, quantitative serum hCG estimations may prove useful. An hCG value of 1000 IU/L represents the cut-off level above which the absence of an intrauterine sac at TVS should raise suspicion of an abnormal pregnancy. This discriminatory level has performed well in the hands of investigators who have used it prospectively in women with suspected ectopic pregnancy (Bree *et al.*, 1989; Cacciatore *et al.*, 1990a; Box 3.2). In these studies, when the hCG level was more than 1000 IU/L, a gestation sac was seen in all intrauterine pregnancies but in none of the ectopic pregnancies; however, the fact that serum hCG levels may remain elevated for several hours after spontaneous abortion means that another measurement should be taken one to two days later if an ectopic pregnancy is suspected in the presence of heavy vaginal bleeding.

In a logical extension of applying these diagnostic tests to symptomatic patients, Cacciatore and colleagues (1994) screened 225 symptom-free pregnant women at increased risk for ectopic pregnancy (based on a history of ectopic pregnancy, tubal or pelvic surgery or pelvic inflammatory disease and current users of intrauterine devices) with TVS and hCG assays. Among 55 (24.4%) women who proved to have an ectopic pregnancy, 46 (84%) of cases were diagnosed at the initial screening at a median of 37 days of gestation and the rest by re-scanning within a few days before complications had occurred. There was a false positive rate of 1.2%. As expected, the initial detection rate was slightly lower in this study than in a previous one from the same group (Cacciatore *et al.*, 1990a) which examined symptomatic patients (84% versus 93%). This is presumably because bleeding within the tube or spillage of blood into the abdominal cavity facilitates detection by TVS in symptomatic patients. Just over 80% of the ectopic pregnancies in the study of Cacciatore *et al.* (1994) could have been diagnosed just by the absence of an intrauterine sac with hCG levels at more than 1000 IU/L, supporting the view that hCG assays supplement TVS in screening for ectopic pregnancy (Grudzinskas and Stabile, 1993).

In conclusion, screening in early high risk pregnancy by TVS and serum hCG assay can reliably diagnose asymptomatic ectopic pregnancies, thus diminishing the likelihood of tubal rupture, haemorrhage and emergency care. This is particularly important in planning optimal surgical treatment for all patients which may reduce the costs (both financial and in terms of personal suffering) associated with emergency treatment. One possible negative aspect of very early diagnosis is enthusiastic overtreatment of ectopic pregnancies which might later resolve spontaneously without complications (Ylostalo *et al.*, 1992); however, prevention of substantial blood loss and tubal rupture is a major benefit, on the basis of which the early screening of at risk groups can be recommended.

6.7   Point summary

1. A gestation sac is seen with TVS 12–14 days after biochemical detection of implantation (hCG more than 10 IU/L). This time interval is longer using TAS.

2. The intrauterine gestation sac is consistently seen when 2–4 mm in diameter (one week after the missed period) when the hCG level is approximately 1000 IU/L (IRP).

3. Up to 70% of patients at risk for ectopic pregnancy have an initial hCG value below the accepted discriminatory level.

4. Any woman with a positive pregnancy test and features suggestive of ectopic pregnancy should have an ultrasound scan.

5. A normal pregnancy at a stage too early to visualise its contents, a failed intrauterine pregnancy or an ectopic gestation may present with an empty sac on TVS.

6. If ultrasound is unhelpful quantitative hCG measurement should be performed. Laparoscopy is indicated if the level is above the discriminatory zone appropriate to the type of ultrasound.

7. Less than a quarter of patients with ectopic pregnancy present with an acute abdomen and evidence of internal bleeding.

8. Only 20% of women with ectopic pregnancy have identifiable risk features. Intrauterine pregnancy is still more likely in this group.

9. Screening in early high risk pregnancy by TVS and serum hCG assay can reliably diagnose asymptomatic ectopic pregnancies, thus preventing tubal rupture, haemorrhage and emergency care.

6.8   References

Atrash, H.K., Friede, A., Hogue, C.J.R. (1987). Ectopic pregnancy mortality in the United States, 1970–1983. *Obstetrics and Gynecology*, **70**: 817–822.

Bree, L.R., Edwards, M., Bohm Velez, M., Beyler, S., Roberts, J., Mendelson, A.B. (1989). Transvaginal sonography in the evaluation of normal early pregnancy: correlation with hCG level. *American Journal of Radiology*, **153**: 75–79.

Cacciatore, B., Stenman, U.H., Ylostalo, P. (1990a) Diagnosis of ectopic pregnancy by vaginal ultrasonography in combination with a discriminatory serum hCG level of 1000 IU/L (IRP). *British Journal Obstetrics and Gynaecology*, **97**: 904–908.

Cacciatore, B., Stenman, U.H., Ylostalo, P. (1994). Early screening for ectopic pregnancy in high-risk symptom-free women. *Lancet*, **343**: 517–518.

Cacciatore, B., Tiitinen, A., Stenman, D.H., Ylostalo, P. (1990b). Normal early pregnancy: serum hCG levels and vaginal ultrasonography findings. *British Journal of Obstetrics and Gynecology*, **97**: 899–903.

DiMarchi, J.M., Josas, T.S., Hale, R.W. (1989). What is the significance of hCG value in ectopic pregnancy? *Obstetrics and Gynecology*, **74**: 851–855.

Fleischer, A.C., Pennell, R.G., McKee, M.S., Worrell, J.A., Keefe, B., Herbert, C.M., Hill, G.A., Cartwright, P.S., Keeple, D.M. (1990). Ectopic pregnancy: features at transvaginal sonography. *Radiology*, **174**: 375–378.

Grudzinskas, J.G., Stabile, I. (1993). Ectopic pregnancy: are biochemical tests at all useful? *British Journal Obstetrics and Gynaecology*, **100**: 510–511.

Hann, L., Bachman, D., McArdle, C. (1984). Co-existent intrauterine and ectopic pregnancy: re-evaluation. *Radiology*, **152**: 151–153.

May, W., Miller, B., Greiss, F.C. (1976). Maternal deaths from ectopic pregnancy in the South Atlantic region. *American Journal of Obstetrics and Gynecology*, **132**: 140–144.

Parvey, H.R., Maklad, N. (1993). Pitfalls in the transvaginal sonographic diagnosis of ectopic pregnancy. *Journal of Ultrasound in Medicine*, **12**: 139–144.

Seppala, M., Purhonen, M. (1987) The use of hCG and other pregnancy proteins in the diagnosis of ectopic pregnancy. *Clinical Obstetrics and Gynecology*, **30**: 148–154.

Soussis, I., Dimitri, E.S., Oskarsson, T., Margara, R., Winston, R. (1991). Diagnosis of ectopic pregnancy by vaginal ultrasonography in combination with a discriminatory serum hCG level of 1000 IU/L.

British Journal of Obstetrics and Gynaecology, **97** (10): 904–908.

Stabile, I., Campbell, S. (1992). Ultrasound diagnosis of spontaneous miscarriage. In: *Spontaneous Abortion: Diagnosis and Treatment*, (eds. I. Stabile, J.G. Grudzinskas, T. Chard), pp. 63–86. Springer-Verlag, London.

Stiller, R.J., de Regt, R.H., Blair, E. (1989). Transvaginal sonography in patients at risk for ectopic pregnancy. *American Journal of Obstetrics and Gynecology*, **161**: 930–933.

Ylostalo, P. , Cacciatore, B., Sjoberg, J., Kaariainen, M., Tenhunen, A., Stenman, U.H. (1992). Expectant management of ectopic pregnancy. *Obstetrics and Gynecology*, **80**: 345–48.

Extratubal and unusual ectopic pregnancies

7.1 Introduction

Approximately 3–5% of all ectopic pregnancies are extratubal. They account for one-fifth of all maternal deaths from ectopic pregnancy. Extratubal implantation occurs most commonly in the ovary, cervix and abdominal cavity. Very rarely the fertilized ovum implants in a rudimentary uterine horn or on the broad ligament. The incidence, clinical features and diagnosis of each of these forms of ectopic pregnancy are described in this chapter.

7.2 Ovarian pregnancy

One to three percent of all ectopic pregnancies are located in the ovary. Ovarian pregnancy occurs when the ovum is fertilised and implants within its follicle (primary) or from implantation of an early tubal abortion on the surface of the ovary (secondary). It occurs in approximately one in 7000 deliveries. Twin ovarian pregnancy has been reported (Ohba *et al.*, 1992). The criteria for surgical diagnosis of ovarian pregnancy are an intact tube on the affected side with the gestation sac located at the ovarian site and connected to the uterus by the utero-ovarian ligament (Box 7.1). In addition, histological evidence of ovarian tissue in the wall of the sac should be obtained (Spiegelberg, 1878). Lehfeldt *et al.* (1970) have shown that users of the intrauterine contraceptive device (IUD) have a higher ratio of ovarian to total ectopic pregnancies (1 : 9) than non-users. The IUD prevents intrauterine implantation in 99.5% of cases, tubal implantation in 95% of cases and ovarian implantation not at all. Primary ovarian pregnancy may occur in the polycystic ovary syndrome (Catalado, 1992) and after *in-vitro* fertilisation (IVF) and embryo transfer (Marcus and Brinsden, 1993).

> **Box 7.1. Surgical/pathological diagnosis of primary ovarian pregnancy (Spiegelberg, 1878).**
>
> - Intact tube on affected side, distinct from the ovary
> - Gestation sac located within the ovary and connected to the uterus by the ovarian ligament
> - Histological evidence of ovarian tissue in the wall of the sac

Clomiphene ovulation induction has been reported to cause heterotopic ovarian pregnancy (De Muylder *et al.*, 1994).

As the pregnancy grows, the chorion ruptures and is extruded from the ovary; because the embryo is in proximity to the tube, the clinical features are similar to those of a tubal pregnancy (Mall and Cullen, 1913). Diagnostic tests such as human chorionic gonadotrophin (hCG) and ultrasonography are no more helpful than in a tubal pregnancy. Rarely, a gestation sac is identified at ultrasonography within the ovary. The exact location of the pregnancy is usually established at laparoscopy (Carter *et al.*, 1993), laparotomy or histology: the preoperative diagnosis is usually tubal pregnancy or an ovarian tumour. Most cases come to surgery by the end of the second trimester (Serreyn *et al.*, 1983). At laparoscopy, the tube is normal but the ovarian pregnancy may be indistinguishable from a ruptured corpus luteum cyst. Treatment is by wedge resection, ovarian cystectomy or, more recently, by laparoscopic laser surgery (Goldenberg *et al.*, 1994). Case reports document successful treatment of ovarian pregnancy with methotrexate (Shamma and Schwartz, 1992; Chelmow *et al.*, 1994; Hirose *et al.*, 1994) or local prostaglandin F2alpha (Koike *et al.*, 1990), but not mifepristone (Levin *et al.*, 1990). Rarely, complications such as uncontrollable haemorrhage necessitate oophorectomy or salpingo-oophorectomy.

7.3   Abdominal pregnancy

Abdominal pregnancy is rare (incidence ranging from one in 3000 to one in 10000 deliveries); it represents approximately 1% of all ectopic pregnancies (Delke *et al.*, 1982). As with a tubal pregnancy, the older, non-white woman with few previous pregnancies who may be infertile (secondary) is at greatest risk of abdominal pregnancy. Early primary abdominal pregnancy after IVF and embryo transfer has been reported (Balmaceda *et al.*, 1993).

Box 7.2. Surgical/pathological diagnosis of primary abdominal pregnancy (Studdiford, 1942).

- Normal tubes and ovaries with no evidence of recent or past injury
- No evidence of uteroplacental fistula
- Pregnancy attached only to peritoneal surface
- Possibility of secondary implantation following primary tubal nidation excluded by the pregnancy occurring early enough in gestation*

*Advanced abdominal pregnancy is considered secondary in origin

---

Abdominal pregnancy may occur as a primary implant or more commonly develop secondary to tubal abortion or rupture. The criteria for diagnosis of primary abdominal pregnancy (Box 7.2) include normal tubes and ovaries with no evidence of a utero–tubal fistula (Studdiford, 1942). Implantation may occur anywhere in the abdominal cavity, but most often occurs on the surface of the pelvic peritoneum or on that of one of the reproductive organs, e.g. after uterine perforation. An abdominal pregnancy may remain undetected; after the fetus dies it becomes a lithopaedion which may be discovered at laparotomy years later. Very rarely, viable intrauterine and abdominal pregnancies may occur simultaneously.

The clinical features of early abdominal pregnancy are indistinguishable from those of a tubal pregnancy. As the pregnancy advances, unexplained abdominal pain, nausea or vomiting may occur. The location of the abdominal pain is related to the site of implantation. Braxton-Hicks contractions are notably absent. Fetal movements may be painful and felt high in the abdomen. Abdominal tenderness is the most consistent finding on examination. In half of all cases the fetal lie is abnormal. On bimanual examination, the uterus is usually normal in size, the cervix may be uneffaced and displaced laterally by the abdominal conceptus. Rarely, the uterus and fetus are felt separate from each other. In advanced pregnancy the fetus may be palpated easily, giving the clinical impression that it lies just under the skin of the abdomen. Suspicion may also be raised when the induction of labour with prostaglandins or oxytocin fails to cause uterine contractions, although this is not universal. Most cases, however, of abdominal pregnancy are discovered at laparotomy, the preoperative diagnosis having been tubal pregnancy or abruption.

Examination under anaesthesia and soft tissue X-ray examination have given way to diagnosis by magnetic resonance imaging (Cohen *et al.*, 1985) and ultrasound (Angtuaco *et al.*, 1994). As pregnancy advances, lateral X-ray studies of the abdomen reveal fetal parts overlapping the

> **Box 7.3. Ultrasound diagnosis of abdominal pregnancy (Allibone** *et al*, 1981).
>
> - Uterus enlarged (8–10 weeks, size) but empty
> - Fetal parts outside the uterus, close to maternal abdominal wall
> - Unusual fetal positions
> - Ectopic placenta which is difficult to outline
> - Absence of uterine wall between fetus and maternal bladder
> - Absence of amniotic fluid between fetal chest or head and placenta

maternal spine in approximately 10% of cases. Ultrasound diagnosis of an early abdominal pregnancy shares the same difficulties as that of a tubal pregnancy. Identification of a small gestation sac among other abdominal organs is almost impossible. Locating the site of implantation may be difficult even with transvaginal sonography (TVS), particularly if the pregnancy is outside the pelvis. In the second trimester, careful ultrasound examination of the fetus may still miss the ectopic location, unless the uterus (empty) is always identified between the fetus and the bladder. Oligohydramnios may further cloud the picture. As the placenta enlarges it may be possible to see it lying attached to an abdominal organ. It is often difficult to delineate (Box 7.3).

The fetal abnormality rate ranges from 35% to 75% (Stafford and Ragan, 1977; Stevens, 1993). In most cases, morphological malformations are caused by pressure in association with severe oligohydramnios. The most frequent malformations are facial asymmetry, talipes and lung hypoplasia (Cartwright *et al*., 1986). Extremely high serum alphafetoprotein levels (Tromans *et al*., 1984) but normal liquor values (Jackson *et al*., 1993) have been reported in abdominal pregnancy.

Management depends on when in the pregnancy the diagnosis is made. In the first and last trimester, laparotomy and surgical removal of the fetus is indicated as soon as the diagnosis is made because of the high associated maternal mortality (up to 20%) and morbidity rates (Delke *et al*., 1982). There have been isolated case reports of preoperative transcatheter embolisation of abdominal pregnancy (Kerr *et al*., 1993).

Blood loss is unpredictable but usually heavy. Surgery must be carried out by the most experienced team member as it may be necessary to resect vital structures involved in the implantation site. This should not begin until sufficient cross-matched blood is available. At laparotomy, the abdomen is first inspected carefully to determine the site of implantation. The sac is opened and the fetus is removed very carefully to avoid disturbing the placenta, which may otherwise lead to uncontrolled bleeding. If the blood supply to the placenta is readily isolated and ligated (e.g. if it is attached to the back of the uterus), it may be safe to remove it. Otherwise it is best to ligate the cord close to its insertion and leave the placenta *in situ*. Marsupialisation of the amniotic cavity by suturing the edges to the peritoneal opening of the abdomen followed by packing it with gauze is recommended by some to prevent the placenta from separating prematurely. The gauze pack is removed gradually in the early postoperative period.

Diagnosis in the second trimester in an asymptomatic patient has prompted some to await fetal viability in the hospital environment. Blood must always be available, as surgery may be needed at any time for massive intraperitoneal haemorrhage, usually from the placenta. If the fetus has died, the operation may also be delayed to await partial resorption of the placenta.

Postoperative complications include secondary haemorrhage, infection and ileus. Haemorrhage occurs because the placenta, if left *in situ*, may separate before vessels at its base have thrombosed. Peritonitis, abscess, fistula formation, wound dehiscence or persistent hydronephrosis (Weiss and Stone, 1994) are possible especially if the placenta is left behind. The risks of leaving the placenta behind have prompted some to consider chemotherapeutic agents such as methotrexate to promote placental resorption (Rahman *et al.*, 1982), although complications actually increased after methotrexate treatment in this preliminary report. The use of the medical anti-gravity suit as described by Sandberg and Pelligra (1983) may improve the prognosis by allowing the surgeon to be more aggressive in his/her attempts to remove the placenta. This is not widely available.

7.4   Intraligamentous pregnancy

An intraligamentous pregnancy develops in the space confined by the anterior and posterior leaves of the broad ligament, by the levator ani inferiorly, by the uterus medially, the pelvic side wall laterally and by the fallopian tube above (Patterson and Grant, 1975). All such pregnancies must be secondary as there is no connection between this space and the peritoneal cavity. Primary implantation in the ovary or peritoneal surface with subsequent rupture and secondary nidation in the intraligamentous space is the likely mechanism of this rare (one in 50000 to one in 180000) form of extraperitoneal abdominal pregnancy.

Abdominal pain is thought to be related to tension or pressure on the peritoneum which surrounds the gestation sac. In one-third of cases the uterus is felt separate from the pregnancy and the cervix is displaced laterally on pelvic examination. In the third trimester an unstable fetal lie is characteristic. Preoperative diagnosis in the first or second trimesters is exceptionally difficult.

The diagnosis is usually made at the time of surgery. The timing, extent and complications of surgery are similar to those of an abdominal pregnancy, except that as the pregnancy is wholly extraperitoneal, torrential haemorrhage is less likely. Problems with extensive placental invasion of nearby structures rarely arise and the placenta can usually be removed in its entirety. Maternal mortality from an intraligamentous pregnancy has fallen because of earlier diagnosis.

7.5   Interstitial pregnancy

A pregnancy which develops in the intramural or cornual portion of the fallopian tube is interstitial. It occurs once in 2500 to 5000 live births and comprises 2–4% of all ectopic pregnancies. Once nidation has occurred, the proximity to the myometrium and prominent vasculature of this most medial part of the fallopian tube encourages development of the pregnancy at this site. For the same reasons, extensive haemorrhage often results in emergency presentation with shock (patients in group 1), typically when the tube ruptures in the second trimester (Felmus and Pedowitz, 1953). Rarely, a secondary abdominal pregnancy results. Predisposing factors are similar to those of other tubal pregnancies, with the notable addition that neither cornual resection at the time of salpingectomy for a tubal pregnancy nor ipsilateral salpingo-oophorectomy protect the patient from a subsequent interstitial pregnancy on the same side.

Sonographic diagnosis late in the first trimester is possible (Smith *et al.*, 1981; Auslender *et al.*, 1983). The sac is located in the lateral part of the uterine fundus and is not entirely surrounded by myometrium. At laparoscopy there may be an asymmetrical swelling on the uterus and the round ligament is medial to it (cf. angular pregnancy). Differential diagnosis from a fibroid uterus is aided by evidence of increased vasculature over the implantation site.

Tubal rupture in the second trimester often involves the adjacent uterus; the uterus should be removed. Treatment options in the first trimester depend to a certain extent on the state of the other tube. If the contralateral tube is healthy, salpingectomy and cornual resection is the treatment of choice. Tubal re-implantation is feasible if the opposite tube is diseased. Tanaka *et al.* (1982) were the first to report the successful use of methotrexate (30 mg intramuscularly on the first day and 15 mg for five days) to treat interstitial ectopic pregnancy. Several case reports followed (Brandes *et al.*, 1986; Fernandez *et al.*, 1991; Karsdorp *et al.*, 1992) using systemic and/or local injection of methotrexate into the pregnancy. A few of these successful cases were viable interstitial pregnancies with hCG levels up to 16800 IU/L (Karsdorp *et al.*, 1992). Others have been less successful (Voigt *et al.*, 1994). This is discussed in greater detail in Chapter 8.

7.6   Cervical pregnancy

A cervical pregnancy is one that implants entirely within the cervical canal. The criteria for surgical/pathological diagnosis are a closed internal os and a partially open external os with the products of conception confined solely to the endocervix. Histologically, cervical glands are identified opposite to the placental site which itself is firmly attached to the endocervix. The placental site is below the peritoneal reflection of the anterior and posterior surfaces of the uterus and there is no trophoblast or fetal parts within the body of the uterus (Rubin, 1911). The reported incidence ranges from one in 2500 to one in 18000 deliveries (0.1% of ectopic pregnancies). In most cases its aetiology is unclear, although the predominant risk factor is reportedly a history of previous curettage (Shinagawa and Nagayama, 1969). This cannot be considered the sole predisposing factor (Ginsburg *et al.*, 1994), as curettage is a commonly performed procedure, whereas cervical pregnancy is very rare. There have been case reports of cervical pregnancy after intrauterine insemination and ovulation induction with clomiphene citrate (Kaplan *et al.*, 1990) or human menopausal gonadotrophin (Balasch *et al.*, 1994) as well as IVF (Weyerman *et al.*, 1989), although a cause and effect relationship is not proven.

The typical patient is an older multigravida in whom sometimes painless vaginal bleeding after amenorrhoea raises the suspicion of an incomplete abortion. The cervix is soft and the external os partly open with the products of conception within the endocervix. Occasionally, heavy bleeding from the cervical implantation, which is refractory to oxytocin, follows uterine evacuation for what was thought to be an incomplete abortion (Box 7.4). Apart from spontaneous abortion, the differential diagnosis includes cervical cancer, placenta praevia, trophob-

---

Box 7.4. Diagnosis of cervical pregnancy.

Clinical
- Expanded dilated cervix with normal sized uterus on vaginal examination
- Products of conception contained entirely within the cervix and below the internal os
- Fractional curettage reveals no products of conception from uterus

Ultrasound
- Enlarged cervix containing the gestation sac
- Empty uterus which is smaller in size than the cervix (the hour-glass appearance)
- Endocervix may only contain indistinct components

---

last tumour and a degenerating cervical fibroid. The ultrasound image is usually diagnostic: the cervix is enlarged and contains the gestation sac which is typically round or oval and may contain a yolk sac and/or a viable fetus. By contrast, the sac in a pregnancy that is aborting spontaneously is more often irregular and usually diminishes in size within a few days. The uterus is empty and smaller in size than the cervix (the hour-glass appearance). Sometimes the endocervix only contains indistinct components, making the distinction from incomplete abortion difficult, unless enlargement of the cervix is noted (Rosenberg and Williamson, 1992; Laughlin *et al.*, 1983). Diagnosis by transvaginal sonography (TVS) is also possible (Rottem *et al.*, 1993; Frates *et al.*, 1994). Early diagnosis and successful non-surgical treatment of a viable combined intrauterine and cervical pregnancy has also been reported (Frates *et al.*, 1994; Peleg *et al.*, 1994).

Most cervical pregnancies abort but a few continue to grow as the isthmus is incorporated into the cervix to accomodate the expanding pregnancy (Marcovici *et al.*, 1994). Rarely, the pregnancy goes to term. Advanced cases are treated by hysterectomy. Modern management of early cases is conservative and includes evacuation of the pregnancy by suction curettage after vascular ligation by cervical cerclage or laterally placed figure of eight sutures. Packing the cervix or using pressure from an inflated Foley catheter is often successful in arresting haemorrhage. Treatment with systemic and local methotrexate (Farabow *et al.*, 1983; Oyer *et al.*, 1988; Wolcott *et al.*, 1988; Kaplan *et al.*, 1990; Balasch *et al.*, 1994; Timor-Tritsch *et al.*, 1994), either alone or in combination with cervical instrumentation, TVS-guided injection of potassium chloride (Frates *et al.*, 1994), oral etoposide (Segna *et al.*, 1990) or intravenous actinomycin D (Brand *et al.*, 1993) has been reported with varying degrees of success. Earlier diagnosis and treatment have lowered the maternal mortality rate of cervical pregnancy to almost nil (Parente *et al.*, 1983). Case reports document successful pregnancy after previous conservative treatment (Frates *et al.*, 1994).

7.7   Cornual pregnancy

A cornual pregnancy (sometimes called rudimentary horn pregnancy) occurs in the atretic horn of a bicornuate uterus. It is very rare (one in 100 000 pregnancies) and carries a 5% maternal mortality rate. Transperitoneal migration of the sperm or fertilised ovum probably occurs as in most cases there is no connection between the two horns (Cohn and Goldenberg, 1976).

Abdominal pain occurs before or with rupture which, in most cases, happens early in the second trimester. A few cases (10%) reach term and 1% deliver a live child (O'Leary and O'Leary, 1963). Pelvic examination in a cornual pregnancy may occasionally reveal an asymmetrical uterus. A few cases are diagnosed pre-operatively by ultrasound (Holden and Hart, 1983).

Unless the fetus is almost mature, treatment is excision of the rudimentary horn and tube on the affected side. A postoperative intravenous pyelogram is recommended to identify possible associated urinary tract abnormalities.

7.8   Angular pregnancy

Despite the similarity in terminology, an angular pregnancy is distinct from a cornual one; although it may occur in an abnormal uterus, both congenital and acquired, the pregnancy is always intrauterine and located medial to the insertion of the fallopian tube. Most cases are asymptomatic; a few present with abdominal pain and vaginal bleeding. A retained placenta may be the only clue to this form of pregnancy. Differential diagnosis from interstitial pregnancy is possible ultrasonically if the myometrium is identified all the way around the gestation sac. Surgically, the two conditions are distinguished by the position of the round ligament, which in an angular pregnancy is inserted lateral to the conceptus.

Few angular pregnancies which develop in a normal uterus will rupture, but many of these pregnancies abort. Approximately a quarter result in a live child. If the fetus is alive, conservative management is recommended (Jansen and Elliott, 1981).

7.9   Intramural pregnancy

It is extremely rare for a pregnancy to implant entirely within the myometrium and to have no contact with the endometrial or fallopian tube cavities. It has been suggested that previous uterine perforation leads to a sinus or passage through which the blastocyst reaches the myometrium (McGowan, 1965).

Abdominal pain is typical and the differential diagnosis from abruption difficult. The diagnosis is made histologically after the ruptured uterus is removed.

7.10   Point summary

1. Approximately 5% of all ectopic pregnancies are extratubal, of which ovarian pregnancy is the least uncommon (one in 7000 deliveries). Although rare, extratubal pregnancies are associated with high maternal morbidity and mortality rates.

2. Ovarian pregnancy accounts for 1–3% of all ectopic pregnancies. Treatment is by wedge resection, cystectomy or oophorectomy.

3. Abdominal pregnancy is treated by laparotomy and surgical removal of the fetus in the first and third trimester. Unless easily removed, the placenta is left *in situ* to avoid catastrophic intraperitoneal haemorrhage.

3. Interstitial pregnancy accounts for 2–4% of all ectopic pregnancies. Extensive haemorrhage often results in emergency presentation with shock.

4. Cervical pregnancy is rare (one in 18 000 deliveries). The key to conservative treatment (suction curettage after cervical cerclage or chemotherapeutic agents) is accurate early diagnosis, usually by ultrasound.

5. Cornual pregnancy occurs in the atretic horn of a bicornuate uterus (one in 100 000 pregnancies). The maternal mortality rate is 5%.

Treatment is by excision of the rudimentary horn and tube on the affected side.

7.11   References

Allibone, G.W., Fagan, C.J., Porter, S.C. (1981). The sonographic features of intraabdominal pregancy. *Journal of Clinical Ultrasound*, **9**: 383–387.

Angtuaco, T.L., Shah, H.R., Neal, M.R., Quirk, J.G. (1994). Ultrasound evaluation of abdominal pregnancy. *Critical Reviews in Diagnostic Imaging*, **35**(1): 1–59.

Auslender, R., Arodi, J., Pascal, B., Abramovici, H. (1983). Interstitial pregnancy: early diagnosis by ultrasonography. *American Journal of Obstetrics and Gynecology*, **146**: 717–718.

Balasch, J., Penarrubia, J., Ballesca, J.L., Creus, M., Casamitjana, R., Vanrell, J.A. (1994). Intrauterine insemination, cervical pregnancy and successful treatment with methotrexate. *Human Reproduction*, **9**(8): 1580–1583.

Balmaceda, J.P., Bernardini, L., Asch, R.H., Stone, S.C. (1993). Early primary abdominal pregnancy after *in-vitro* fertilization and embryo transfer. *Journal of Reproduction and Genetics*, **10**(4): 317–320.

Brand, E., Gibbs, R.S., Davidson, S.A. (1993). Advanced cervical pregnancy treated with actinomycin D. *British Journal of Obstetrics and Gynaecology*, **100**(5): 491–2.

Brandes, M.C, Youngs, D.D., Goldstein, D.P., Parmley, T.H. (1986). Treatment of cornual pregnancy with methotrexate. *American Journal of Obstetrics and Gynecology*, **155**: 655–657.

Carter, J.E., Ekuan, J., Kallins G.J. (1993). Laparoscopic diagnosis and excision of an intact ovarian pregnancy. A case report. *Journal of Reproductive Medicine*, **38**(12): 962–963.

Cartwright, P.S., Brown, J.E., David, R.J. (1986). Advanced abdominal pregnancy associated with fetal pulmonary hypoplasia: report of a case. *American Journal of Obstetrics and Gynecology*, **155**: 396–397.

Cataldo, N.A. (1992). Ovarian pregnancy in polycystic ovary syndrome: a case report. *International Journal of Fertility*, **37**(3): 144–145.

Chelmow, D., Gates, E., Penzias, A.S. (1994). Laparoscopic diagnosis and methotrexate treatment of an ovarian pregnancy: a case report. *Fertility and Sterility*, **62**(4): 879–881.

Cohen, J.M., Weinreb, J.C., Lowe, T.W., Brown, C. (1985). MR imaging of a viable full-term abdominal pregnancy. *American Journal of Radiology*, **145**: 407–408.

Cohn, F.L., Goldenberg, R.L (1976). Term pregnancy in an unattached rudimentary uterine horn. *Obstetrics and Gynecology*, **48**: 234–236.

Delke, I., Veridiano, N.P., Tancer, M.L. (1982). Abdominal pregnancy: review and current management and addition of ten cases. *Obstetrics and Gynecology*, **60**: 200–204.

De Muylder, X., De Loecker, P., Campo, R. (1994). Heterotopic ovarian pregnancy after clomiphene ovulation induction. *European Journal of Obstetrics, Gynecology and Reproductive Biology*, **53**(1): 65–66.

Farabow, W.S., Fulton, J.W., Fletcher Jr, V (1983). Cervical pregnancy treated with methotrexate. *North Carolina Medical Journal*, **44**: 91–93.

Felmus, L.B., Pedowitz, P. (1953), Interstitial pregnancy. A survey of 45 cases. *American Journal of Obstetrics and Gynecology*, **166**: 1271–1279.

Fernandez, H., DeZiegler, D., Bourget, P., Feltain, P., Frydman, R. (1991). The place of methotrexate in the managemnet of interstitial pregnancy. *Human Reproduction*, **6**: 302–306.

Frates, M.C., Benson, C.B., Doubilet, P.M., Di Salvo, D.N., Brown, D.L., Laing, F.C., Rein, M.S., Osathanondh, R. (1994). Cervical ectopic pregnancy: results of conservative treatment. *Radiology*, **191**(3): 773–775.

Ginsburg, E.S., Frates, M.C., Rein, M.S., Fox, J.H., Hornstein, M.D., Friedman, A.J. (1994). Early diagnosis and treatment of cervical pregnancy in an *in-vitro* fertilization program. *Fertility and Sterility*, **61**(5): 966–969.

Goldenberg, M., Bider, D., Mashiach, S., Rabinovici, J., Dulitzky, M., Oelsner, G. (1994). Laparoscopic laser surgery of primary ovarian pregnancy. *Human Reproduction*, **9**(7): 1337–1338.

Hirose, M., Nomura, T., Wakuda, K., Ishiguro, T., Yoshida, Y. (1994). Combined intrauterine and ovarian pregnancy: a case report. *Asia Oceania Journal of Obstetrics and Gynaecology*, **20** (1): 25–29.

Holden, R., Hart, P. (1983). First trimester rudimentary horn pregnancy: pre-rupture ultrasound diagnosis. *Obstetrics and Gynecology*, **61**: 56s–58s.

Jackson, S., Hollingworth, T., Macpherson, M. (1993). Elevated serum alpha fetoprotein and normal liquor alpha fetoprotein values in association with an abdominal pregnancy. *Australian and New Zealand Journal of Obstetrics and Gynaecology*, **33**(2): 214–215.

Jansen, R.P.S., Elliott, P.M. (1981). Angular intrauterine pregnancy. *Obstetrics and Gynecology*, **58**: 167–175.

Kaplan, B.R., Brandt, T., Javaheri, G., Scommegna, A. (1990). Non-surgical treatment of a viable cervical pregnancy with intra-amniotic methotrexate. *Fertility and Sterility*, **53**: 941–943.

Karsdorp, V.H.M., van der Veen, F., Schats, R., Boer-Meisel, M.E., Kenemans, P. (1992). Successful treatment with methotrexate of five vital interstitial pregnancies. *Human Reproduction*, **7**: 1164–1169.

Kerr, A., Trambert, J., Mikhail, M., Hodges, L., Runowicz, C. (1993).

Preoperative transcatheter embolization of abdominal pregnancy: report of three cases. *Journal of Vascular Interventional Radiology*, **4**(6): 733–735.

Koike, H., Chuganji, Y., Watanabe, H., Kaneko, M., Noda, S., Mori, N. (1990). Conservative treatment of ovarian pregnancy by local prostaglandin F2alpha injection. *American Journal of Obstetrics and Gynecology*, **163**: 696 (letter).

Laughlin, C.L., Lee, T.G., Richards, R.C., (1983). Ultrasonographic diagnosis of cervical ectopic pregnancy. *Journal of Ultrasound in Medicine*, **2**: 137–139.

Lehfeldt, H., Tietze, C., Gorsterin, F. (1970). Ovarian pregnancy and the intrauterine device. *American Journal of Obstetrics and Gynecology*, **108**: 1005–1009.

Levin. J.H., Maria Lacarra, R.N., d'Ablaing, G., Grimes, D.A., Vermesh, M. (1990). Mifepristone (RU 486) failure in an ovarian heterotopic pregnancy. *American Journal of Obstetrics and Gynecology*, **163**: 543–544.

McGowan, L. (1965) Intramural pregnancy. *Journal of the American Medical Association*, **192**: 637–638.

Mall, C., Cullen, E.K. (1913). Ovarian pregnancy located in the graafian follicle. *Surgery Gynecology Obstetrics*, **17**: 698–701.

Marcovici, I., Rosenzweig, B.A., Brill, A.I., Khan, M., Scommegna, A. (1994). Cervical pregnancy: case reports and a current literature review. *Obstetrics and Gynecological Survey*, **49**(1): 49–55.

Marcus, S.F., Brinsden, P.R. (1993). Primary ovarian pregnancy after *in-vitro* fertilization and embryo transfer: report of seven cases. *Fertility and Sterility*, **60**(1): 167–169.

Ohba, T., Miyazaki, K., Kouno, T., Okamura, H. (1992). Ovarian twin pregnancy. *Acta Obstetrica Gynecologica Scandinavica*, **71**(4): 305–307.

O'Leary, J.L., O'Leary, J.A. (1963). Rudimentary horn pregnancy. *Obstetrics and Gynecology*, **22**: 371–375.

Oyer, R., Tarakjian, D., Lev-Toaff, A. (1988). Treatment of cervical pregnancy with methotrexate. *Obstetrics and Gynecology*, **71**: 469–471.

Parente, J.T., Chau-Su, O., Levy, J., Legatt, E. (1983). Cervical pregnancy analysis: a review and report of five cases. *Obstetrics and Gynecology*, **62**: 79–82.

Patterson, W.G., Grant, K.A. (1975). Advanced intraligamentous pregnancy. *Obstetrics and Gynecological Survey*, **30**: 715–726.

Peleg, D., Bar-Hava, I., Neuman-Levin, M., Ashkenazi, J., Ben-Rafael, Z. (1994). Early diagnosis and successful non-surgical treatment of viable combined intrauterine and cervical pregnancy. *Fertility and Sterility*, **62**(2): 405–408.

Rahman, M.S., Al-Suleiman, S.A., Rahman, J., Al-Sibai, M.H. (1982). Advanced abdominal pregnancy: observation in 10 cases. *Obstetrics and Gynecology*, **59**: 366–372.

Rosenberg, R.D., Williamson, M.R. (1992). Cervical ectopic pregnancy: avoiding pitfalls in the ultrasonographic diagnosis. *Journal of Ultrasound in Medicine*, **11**(7): 365–367.

Rottem, S., Timor-Tritsch, I.L., Thaler, I. (1993). Assessment of pelvic pathology by high frequency transvaginal sonography. In: *Ultrasound in Obstetrics and Gynecology*, (eds F. Chervenak, G.C. Isaacson, S. Campbell,) pp 1629–1641. Little, Brown and Company, Boston.

Rubin, I.C. (1911). Cervical pregnancy. *Surgery, Gynecology and Obstetrics*, **13**: 625–628.

Sandberg, E.C., Pelligra, R. (1983). The medical anti-gravity suit for management of surgically uncontrollable bleeding associated with abdominal pregnancy. *American Journal of Obstetrics and Gynecology*, **146**: 519–525.

Segna, R.A., Mitchell, D.R., Misas, J.E. (1990). Successful treatment of cervical pregnancy with oral etoposide. *Obstetrics and Gynecology*, **76**: 945–947.

Serreyn, R., Kermans, G., Cuvelier, C. (1983). Unruptured primary ovarian pregnancy. *Archives of Gynecology*, **234**: 153–157.

Shamma, F.N., Schwartz, L.B. (1992). Primary ovarian pregnancy successfully treated with methotrexate. *American Journal of Obstetrics and Gynecology*, **167**: 1307–1308.

Shinagawa, S., Nagayama, M. (1969). Cervical pregnancy as a possible sequela of induced abortion. *American Journal of Obstetrics and Gynecology*, **105**: 282–283.

Smith, H.J., Hanken, H., Brundelet, P.J. (1981). Ultrasound diagnosis of interstitial pregnancy. *Acta Obstetrica Gynecologica Scandinavia*, **60**: 413–415.

Spiegelberg, O. (1878). Zur casuistik der ovarialschwangerschaft. *Archives Gynaekology*, **13**: 73–77.

Stafford, I.C., Ragan, W.D. (1977). Abdominal pregnancy. Review of current management. *Obstetrics and Gynecology*, **50**: 548–552.

Stevens, C.A. (1993). Malformations and deformations in abdominal pregnancy. *American Journal of Medical Genetics*, **47**(8): 1189–1195.

Studdiford, W.E. (1942). Primary peritoneal pregnancy. *American Journal of Obstetrics and Gynecology*, **44**: 487–490.

Tanaka, T., Hayashi, H., Kutsuzawa, T., Fujimoto, S., Ichinoe, K. (1982). Treatment of interstitial ectopic pregnancy with methotrexate: report of a successful case. *Fertility and Sterility*, **37**: 851–852.

Timor-Tritsch, I.E., Monteagudo, A., Mandeville, E.O., Peisner, D.B., Anaya, G.P., Pirrone, E.C. (1994). Successful management of viable cervical pregnancy by local injection of methotrexate guided by transvaginal ultrasonography. *American Journal of Obstetrics and Gynecology*, **170**(3): 737–739.

Tromans, P.P., Coulson, R., Lobb, M.O., Abdulla, U. (1984). Abdominal pregnancy associated with extremely elevated serum alphafetoprotein. Case report. *British Journal of Obstetrics and Gynaecology*, **91**: 296–298.

Voigt, R.R., van der Veen, F., Karsdorp, V.H.M., Hogerzeil, H.V., Ketting, B.W. (1994). Treatment of interstitial pregnancy with methotrexate: report of an unsuccessful case. *Human Reproduction*, **9**(8): 1576–1579.

Weiss, R.E., Stone, N.N. (1994). Persistent maternal hydronephrosis after intra-abdominal pregnancy. *Journal of Urology*, **152**(4): 1196–1198.

Weyerman, P.C., Verhoeven, A.T.M., Alberda, A.T. (1989). Cervical pregnancy after *in-vitro* fertilization and embryo transfer. *American Journal of Obstetrics and Gynecology*, **161**: 1145–1146.

Wolcott, H.D., Kaunitz, A.M., Nuss, R.C (1988). Successful pregnancy after previous conservative treatment of an advanced cervical pregnancy. *Obstetrics and Gynecology*, **71**: 1023–1025.

CHAPTER 8

Medical treatment of ectopic pregnancy

8.1   Introduction

It is thought that up to a quarter of all ectopic pregnancies may be suitable for non-surgical management. Medical treatment of an ectopic pregnancy with systemic (e.g. methotrexate, actinomycin D) or local administration of drugs (e.g. potassium chloride, methotrexate, mifepristone or prostaglandin E2 and F2 alpha) into the gestation sac, has recently been introduced into clinical practice. Unlike surgical treatment, the conceptus is left in the fallopian tube to be spontaneously absorbed. This chapter will describe the indications and complications of this novel therapeutic approach.

8.2   Indications: choice of patients

8.2.1   NON-TUBAL PREGNANCY

The initial report (Tanaka *et al.*, 1982) described the successful use of methotrexate in the treatment of a case of interstitial ectopic pregnancy. The choice of the anti-metabolite methotrexate (which inhibits dihydrofolate reductase and hence stops trophoblastic cell growth), as a first line chemotherapeutic agent is a logical one, in view of extensive experience in its use in the treatment of gestational trophoblastic disease. The addition of folinic acid acts as a rescue to the methotrexate, increasing the effectiveness and safety of the treatment. Three years after the initial report of treatment of a non-tubal ectopic pregnancy with methotrexate, Chotiner (1985) described the successful medical treatment of a tubal pregnancy associated with the severe hyperstimulation syndrome following ovulation induction with menopausal gonadotrophin. The indications for methotrexate treatment and the disadvantages of

---

Box 8.1. Indications for methotrexate and disadvantages of surgery in the treatment of ectopic pregnancy.

Indications	*Disadvantages of surgery*
Cervical pregnancy	Extensive haemorrhage
Interstitial pregnancy	Tubal obstruction and infertility
Ectopic pregnancy and hyperstimulation syndrome	
Persistent trophoblast in ampullary pregnancy after conservative treatment	Further tubal damage
Unruptured tubal ectopic pregnancy	As an alternative to standard conservative surgical techniques

---

surgery in the treatment of different forms of ectopic pregnancy as reported in the literature are listed in Box 8.1.

8.2.2   TUBAL ECTOPIC PREGNANCY

Several case reports followed the original paper by Chotiner (Ory *et al.*,1986; Sauer *et al.*, 1987; Fernandez *et al.*, 1988; Feichtinger and Kemeter, 1989; Groutz *et al.*, 1993). They have clearly shown that the key to success using medical therapy is the selection of patients on the basis of features such as the size of the pregnancy (ideally less than 4 cm), an unruptured tube without active bleeding, serum human chorionic gonadotrophin (hCG) levels of less than 1500 IU/L and a sonographically non-viable pregnancy. Serum progesterone levels after the procedure are variable (Vermesh *et al.*, 1988), but low levels (less than 10 ng/ml) predict more rapid resolution (Ransom *et al.*, 1994). Some have advocated ablation of the corpus luteum during conservative treatment of an ectopic pregnancy to minimise luteal support of the trophoblast (Lindblom *et al.*, 1987). Patients are typically discharged following 3 days of progressive decline in beta hCG levels.

8.2.3   PERSISTENT ECTOPIC PREGNANCY

The other situation in which chemotherapeutic agents may be used is for the treatment of persistent ectopic pregnancy (defined as incomplete removal of ectopic trophoblastic tissue) after conservative surgery

(Higgins and Schwartz, 1986; Cowan *et al.*, 1986; DiMarchi and Cyka, 1992; Parker and Thompson, 1994). The incidence of this complication varies between 0 and 20% after laparoscopy (Vermesh *et al.*,1988) and 0 to 5% after laparotomy (DiMarchi *et al.*, 1987). The literature is replete with case reports of small numbers of patients with this condition treated by repeat surgery, either salpingectomy or salpingostomy (Pouly *et al.*, 1986; Vermesh *et al.*, 1988; Seifer *et al.*, 1993), low dose, i.e. 10–20 mg for five days, oral or parenteral methotrexate (Patsner and Keninsgerg, 1988; Bengtsson *et al.*, 1992; Hoppe *et al.*, 1994), methotrexate and RU486 (Keningsberg *et al.*, 1987) or expectant management alone (DiMarchi *et al.*, 1987). The advantage of medical treatment in this situation is first, the diagnosis has already been confirmed at surgery and, second, the protocol is simple and highly effective, although the risk of delayed haemorrhage necessitates close surveillance in this situation (Dumesic and Hafez, 1991).

8.3   Choice of drug

Methotrexate with citrovorum rescue has been used most widely but actinomycin D, mifepristone, potassium chloride, adrenaline, hypertonic glucose and prostaglandin E2 and F2 alpha each have their proponents and opponents. At present it is difficult to recommend one drug over the other, although the little information that is available suggests that the anti-progesterone RU-486 is less effective than methotrexate (Paris *et al.*, 1986; Keningsberg *et al.*, 1987). The advantage of local treatments such as potassium chloride or hyperosmolar glucose is that they are directed at the ectopic pregnancy, without the systemic side effects of chemo-therapeutic agents (Robertson *et al.*, 1987; Lang *et al.*, 1989). Moreover, local injection into the sac under transvaginal ultrasound (TVS) control can be performed on an outpatient basis without anaesthesia. Potassium chloride has a proven safety and track record in the reduction of multifetal pregnancies (Lynch *et al.*, 1990).

8.4   Dosage and routes of administration

Tubal ectopic pregnancy was initially treated medically via the systemic route. The first reports used 1 mg intramuscular or intravenous methotrexate/kg and 0.1 mg leucovorin/kg (citrovorum rescue) on alternate days for four days to minimise toxicity (Ory *et al.*, 1986; Rodi *et*

Box 8.2. Medical complications of the chemotherapeutic agents used in the treatment of ectopic pregnancy.

Drug	Complications
Methotrexate	Stomatitis, gastritis, pneumonitis, anaemia, hepatic, renal and myelotoxicity
Actinomycin D	Nausea, vomiting, stomatitis, leucopenia, alopecia, aplastic anaemia
Mifepristone	Malaise, nausea, vomiting, rashes, uterine pain
Prostaglandin E2 and F2 alpha	Cardiac arrhythmia, pulmonary oedema, abdominal discomfort
Hypertonic glucose	Venous irritation and thrombophlebitis (i.v. only)
Potassium Chloride	Nausea, vomiting, cardiac and respiratory depression

Box 8.3. Disadvantages of systemic methotrexate as first line treatment of ectopic pregnancy.

- Patient must undergo two potentially risky procedures (anaesthesia and surgery followed by cytotoxic therapy)
- Long-term effects on offspring cannot be excluded on the basis of the available data (Section 8.6)
- Uncertain fertility prospects
- Treatment with a cytotoxic agent requires extensive communication with patients and hospital staff

al., 1986; Sauer *et al.*, 1987; Stovall *et al.*, 1991b). More recently, 50 mg methotrexate/m^2 by single intramuscular injection has been used successfully (Hoppe *et al.*,1994; Ransom *et al.*, 1994). The major disadvantage of parenteral therapy is the risk of systemic toxicity (Box 8.2) which is reduced but not abolished by adding citrovorum rescue to the regimen. Compared to the multidose protocol, the single dose regimen is said to improve patient compliance, reduce the overall cost of treatment and minimise the likelihood of side-effects (Ransom *et al.*, 1994). The use of systemic methotrexate as first line therapy, however, is thought by some (Bengtsson *et al.*, 1992) to be problematic (Box 8.3).

The alternative is to use sonographic or laparoscopic-directed aspiration and/or local injection into the gestation sac. This has been attempted with varying degrees of success (Feichtinger and Kemeter, 1987; Lindblom *et al.*, 1987; Timor-Tritsch *et al.*, 1989; Lang *et al.*, 1990; Lindblom *et al.*, 1990; Fernandez *et al.*, 1993; Parker and Thompson, 1994). The major advantage of local injection into the tube is that a smaller dose (10–15 mg) of methotrexate is sufficient (Kojima *et al.*, 1990). Recently, the administration of these medications by transcervical tubal cannulation under sonographic control has also been performed (Risquez *et al.*, 1990 1992a,b). The technique of transcervical catheterisation is described in Section 8.5.

The protocols for local treatment vary widely. Some have used direct laparoscopic injection of 12.5 mg methotrexate into the ectopic sac, followed 24 hours later by intramuscular methotrexate (0.5 mg/kg of body weight) and folinic acid (0.1 mg/kg of body weight) for five days (Zakut *et al.*, 1989). Others inject a larger dose (50 mg) into the tube, but do not add parenteral therapy (Groutz *et al.*, 1993). Eckford and Fox (1993) reported injecting 0.5 mg 15-methylprostaglandin F2 alpha diluted in 10 ml of saline into the tube; cardiovascular side-effects and abdominal discomfort are more common when higher doses are used (Egarter and Husslein, 1988).

8.5   Techniques

Those with experience in TVS-directed biopsy (e.g. for egg collection in *in-vitro* fertilisation) will have no difficulty in understanding the simplicity of this procedure (Figure 8.1). Details are found in several available textbooks (Timor-Tritsch and Rottem, 1987; Fleischer and Kepple, 1992; Chervenak *et al*, 1993), to which the interested reader is encouraged to refer. If the gestation sac can be accurately identified transvaginally, this is the preferred route by those familiar with needling techniques (Menard *et al.*, 1991). Unfortunately, this is not always possible; indeed, even in the best of hands, TVS may be normal in up to a quarter of patients with ectopic pregnancy (Russell *et al.*, 1993). Similarly, enthusiasts of laparoscopic surgery will probably prefer this route, although the procedure requires general anaesthesia. The needle is usually 10–15 cm long and is injected with care to avoid leakage at the site directly into the gestation sac (Figure 8.1).

Risquez *et al.* (1990) were the first to report selective tubal cannulation allowing non-operative access to the fallopian tube through the vagina and

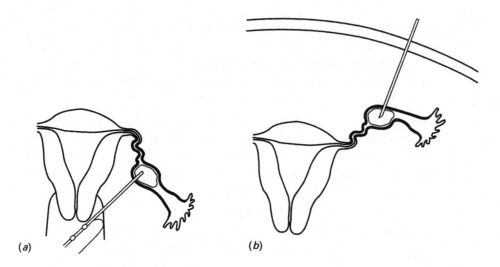

(a)   (b)

Figure 8.1 Diagrammatic representation of (*a*) transvaginal and (*b*) laparoscopic needling of an ectopic pregnancy.

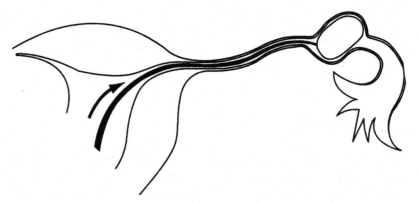

Figure 8.2 Diagrammatic representation of transcervical tubal cannulation.

cervix. The catheter is guided by tactile impression (Figure 8.2) and its correct placement is verified by injecting contrast medium (fluoroscopy) or using ultrasound. Direct visualisation of the ectopic sac is possible followed by intraluminal administration of low dose methotrexate. As there is no needling of the tube, there is less risk of traumatic injury to the vessels. The future of this field lies in progress in fibreoptic technology. Exciting results are awaited.

8.6   Complications

Most of the early literature consisted of case reports (Ichinoe *et al.*, 1987; Shapiro, 1987) describing the indications, dosage and expected adverse reactions of the various therapeutic regimens available. Notable risks include haemosalpinx (Frishman and Seifer, 1993) and pneumonitis, even when the drug (12.5 mg) is injected intra-amniotically (Schoenfeld *et al.*, 1992). A larger retrospective review has shown that up to a third of patients treated with single dose methotrexate experience systemic side-effects such as nausea, diarrhoea or oral irritation (Glock *et al.*, 1994). Prospective randomised controlled studies comparing the various therapeutic modalities are discussed in Section 8.7 (Lang *et al.*, 1990; Fernandez *et al.*, 1991; Risquez *et al.*, 1992a; O'Shea *et al.*, 1994).

The medical complications of the chemotherapeutic agents in use today are listed in Box 8.2. Other dermatological and gynaecological uses of methotrexate have demonstrated that this cytotoxic agent is not associated with congenital abnormalities in subsequent pregnancies (Walden and Bagshaw, 1976) or with an increased risk of malignancy in later life (Bailin *et al.*, 1975). More data is however required before this potential complication is dismissed as insignificant (Ichinoe *et al.*, 1987).

Serial hCG monitoring after medical, expectant and conservative surgical treatment is the rule, although it is uncertain how the results should be interpreted. For example, it has been shown that hCG titres continue to rise for up to one week after local intra-amniotic injection of methotrexate into intact tubal pregnancies (Fernandez *et al.*, 1993; Groutz *et al.*, 1993). hCG levels return to pre-treatment values within 26 $+/-$ ten days (range 10–75 days). This also occurs when methotrexate is administered systemically (Kooi and Kock, 1990; Stovall *et al.*, 1991a). The precise reason for this observation is uncertain. It is possible that exposure to methotrexate can increase the release of hCG from degenerating trophoblast cells or it may be secondary to trauma exerted by the needle puncture itself. Others suggest that it may result from failure of methotrexate therapy because of technical problems such as leakage of methotrexate from the injection sites or inadvertent injection of loci distant from the pregnancy site (Pansky *et al.*, 1992; Zakut *et al.*, 1989). Hence, rising beta hCG titres following methotrexate treatment do not always indicate treatment failure, and no additional treatment is required provided the patient is clinically stable. Similarly, one should not equate undetectable, low or declining beta hCG levels with resolution of the ectopic pregnancy, without taking the whole clinical picture into account. Tulandi *et al.* (1991) have reported that rupture of the ectopic is still possible in such women. They speculate that by distorting tubal anatomy, intratubal bleeding predisposes to tubal rupture.

One final observation concerns the increased pain reported in up to one-third of patients after single dose systemic methotrexate (Glock *et al.*,1994). This is not necessarily an indication for surgical treatment; it may represent tubal abortion or degeneration of the ectopic secondary to the methotrexate. Clearly, each case should be evaluated on its own merits: unstable haematocrit or signs of peritoneal irritation warrant laparoscopy.

8.7   Success rate

Tulandi (1992) has raised the question of 'what is success'? For practical purposes, the term 'complete resolution' can be applied when the serum beta hCG level reaches undetectable levels, the affected tube has returned to normal (as seen by TVS) and no further intervention is required. Analysis of the results of medical treatment using these criteria reveals that most treatments have very similar success rates of 80–95%. This is hardly surprising as the selection criteria for the various forms of medical treatment available are very similar. Others have reported that the failure rate may be closer to 30% (Kooi and Kock, 1992; Ransom *et al.*, 1994).

It may not be valid to pool data from various studies and make comparisons between different investigations, but in the absence of large randomised trials, it may provide some useful information. Lindblom (1993) compared the results of laparoscopically-guided and ultrasound-guided local injection therapy in unruptured tubal pregnancy. Laparoscopically-guided injections had a 93% success rate (117 of 127 cases pooled from seven studies) compared with a 72% success rate for ultrasound-guided injection (49 of 68 cases pooled from five studies).

So far, only five small randomised controlled trials comparing various treatment modalities have been reported, one of which was not completed (Mottla *et al.*, 1992). Lang *et al.* (1990) compared hyperosmolar glucose and PGF2 alpha injection into the tube demonstrating similar success rates in both groups (total of 29 cases). Fernandez *et al.* (1991) compared methotrexate with prostaglandin sulprostone by combined transvaginal and systemic administration, again with similar success rates in each group (total of 14 cases). Mottla *et al.* (1992) began a randomised controlled trial comparing intratubal injection of methotrexate (12.5–25 mg) under laparoscopic control ($n = 7$) with laparoscopic salpingoscopy ($n = 5$), but discontinued it because of poor results in the injection group, although these might have been due to the relatively small dose of methotrexate used.

O'Shea *et al.* (1994) reported the first prospective randomised trial of intra-amniotic methotrexate versus CO_2 laser laparoscopic salpingotomy in the management of 53 unruptured tubal ectopic pregnancies. The two groups were equivalent as far as age, parity, ectopic size, hCG levels and failure rates (12% for laparoscopic salpingotomy and 10% for methotrexate) were concerned. Tubal damage, as demonstrated by hysterosalpingography, was similar in both groups, although long-term pregnancy follow-up was not reported. The authors conclude that tubal pregnancy can be safely and effectively managed either by intra-amniotic methotrexate or laparoscopic salpingotomy. Larger prospective studies are awaited.

Risquez *et al.* (1992a) reported a prospective multicentre trial to examine the efficacy of transcervical tubal cannulation and intraluminal methotrexate injection for the management of tubal ectopic pregnancy. Patients underwent transcervical tubal cannulation under fluoroscopic or ultrasound control and local injection of methotrexate (up to 50 mg). There was complete resolution of the ectopic in 27 of 31 cases (87%). The authors concluded that transcervical tubal catheterization in patients with tubal pregnancies is feasible and can be performed without anaesthesia or analgesia in most cases.

8.8   Subsequent reproductive performance

Having defined success (Section 8.7), the important issue becomes how to measure the outcome of success. The intrauterine pregnancy rate after systemic methotrexate is almost 90% with a recurrent ectopic pregnancy rate of 11% (Stovall *et al.*, 1991b). These short-term results are very similar to those after laparoscopic surgical removal (Pouly *et al.*, 1991). Of greater importance is the long-term outcome, i.e. tubal patency rate and live birth rate.

Tubal patency has been demonstrated by hysterosalpingography (HSG) following methotrexate treatment of an interstitial pregnancy (Tanaka *et al.*, 1982); in four of seven patients with tubal pregnancy treated with systemic methotrexate, one of whom had a subsequent intrauterine pregnancy (Rodi *et al.*, 1986); in seven of ten women with tubal pregnancy successfully treated by injection of methotrexate into the gestation sac under direct laparoscopic vision, one of whom had a successful pregnancy thereafter (Zakut *et al.*, 1989). These small studies suggest that at least two-thirds of women receiving medical treatment for unruptured tubal pregnancy have patent tubes after the procedure.

More recent studies have reported the number of patients who subsequently conceive and go on to have a successful intrauterine pregnancy. One half of the 30 infertile patients successfully treated with 50 mg intramuscular methotrexate/m^2 were desirous of pregnancy, three of whom (with HSG demonstrated bilateral tubal patency) conceived (20%) resulting in three term deliveries and two spontaneous abortions after 2 to 24 months follow-up (Glock *et al.*, 1994). By contrast, Stovall and Ling (1993) reported a conception rate of almost 80% and an intrauterine pregnancy rate of 70% in their group of 120 patients treated with single dose methotrexate. This dramatic difference is most probably related to the fact that a history of infertility (as noted in the study of Glock) is the single most important predictor of poor fertility performance after an ectopic pregnancy (Ory *et al.*, 1993).

Fourteen of 27 patients treated successfully by transcervical cannulation and intraluminal injection of methotrexate were desirous of pregnancy and available for follow-up to assess the return of reproductive potential (Risquez *et al.*, 1992a). All seven patients who subsequently underwent HSG had patency of the affected tube, five of whom later had an intrauterine pregnancy. This approach offers a new alternative for the treatment of selected patients with tubal ectopic pregnancy. Clearly, larger data sets are required to answer the question of whether the reproductive outcome is better after medical or surgical treatment of ectopic pregnancy.

8.9   Which treatment should I use?

It is difficult to choose between the treatment options available. In general, local injection therapy (e.g. methotrexate or potassium chloride) may be superior because of its simplicity, requiring only basic laparoscopic or transvaginal sonographic skills (however, the latter may not be widely available). By contrast, laparoscopic micro-operative procedures typically require greater technical skill. The advantage of the sonographic technique is that general anaesthesia is not required, but this may be countered by the risk of accidental puncture of the blood vessels. It would seem logical that when laparoscopy is needed for diagnosis that laparoscopic-directed tubal injection or conservative surgery should be the treatment of choice, whereas if the diagnosis is made by TVS,

TVS-directed local injection into the ectopic or systemic chemotherapy should be the options. In other words, in the absence of data from large randomised controlled trials, the treatment of choice most probably depends on how the diagnosis is made. This explains why first line treatment with systemic methotrexate is unusual (except in private practice), unless surgery or anaesthesia is contraindicated.

Creinin and Washington (1993) have calculated potential annual cost savings of $265 million in the USA if methotrexate is used in only 30% of patients with ectopic pregnancy with a 90% success rate. From a financial point of view, patients managed by intramuscular methotrexate alone tend to stay in hospital longer than those initially treated with direct injection into the ectopic (Ory *et al.*, 1986; Ichinoe *et al.*, 1987). The potential benefit, however, from shorter inpatient care is at the expense of a greater risk of secondary haemorrhage, at least if laparoscopic intratubal injection of prostaglandin is used (Eckford and Fox, 1993).

In conclusion, tubal pregnancy can be safely and effectively managed either by intra-amniotic chemotherapy (administered laparoscopically or transvaginally) or laparoscopic salpingotomy. There is little to choose between the various drug options available. It should be emphasised that only those centres with access to quantitative hCG and good ultrasound should be using one of these novel treatment modalities. Which one to use depends to a certain extent on personal choice and practical skills, until such time as larger controlled randomised prospective studies indicate which technique is superior in terms of adverse reactions and effects on future fertility.

8.10 Point summary

1. Up to 25% of all ectopic pregnancies may be suitable for non-surgical management.

2. Ectopic pregnancy may be treated medically with systemic methotrexate or by local injection of drugs into the gestation sac, either laparoscopically, transvaginally or by transcervical tubal cannulation.

3. Patients are chosen on the basis of the size of the pregnancy (less than 4 cm), an unruptured tube without active bleeding, serum hCG levels of less than 1500 IU/L and a sonographically non-viable pregnancy.

4. The success rate of medical treatment is 80–90%; approximately two-thirds have patent tubes after the procedure.

5. In the absence of a history of infertility, the subsequent conception

rate is 80% and the recurrent ectopic pregnancy rate is 11%. There is insufficient data concerning the live birth rate of subsequent pregnancies after medical treatment.

8.11   References

Bailin, P.L., Tindall, J.P., Roenigk, H.H., Hogan, M.D. (1975). Is methotrexate therapy for psoriasis carcinogenic? A modified retrospective-prospective analysis. *Journal of the American Medical Association*, **232**: 359–362.

Bengtsson, G., Bryman, I., Thorburn, J., Lindblom, B. (1992). Low-dose oral methotrexate as second line therapy for persistent trophoblast after conservative treatment of ectopic pregnancy. *Obstetrics and Gynecology*, **79**(4): 589–91.

Chervenak, F., Isaacson, G.C., Campbell, S. (1993). *Ultrasound in Obstetrics and Gynecology*. Little Brown and Company, Boston.

Chotiner, H.C. (1985). Non surgical treatment of ectopic pregnancy associated with severe hyperstimulation syndrome. *Obstetrics and Gynecology*, **66**: 740–742.

Cowan, B.D., McGehee, R.P., Bates, G.W. (1986). Treatment of persistent ectopic pregnancy with methotrexate and leukovorum rescue: a case report. *Obstetrics and Gynecology*, **67**: 50s–51s.

Creinin, M.D., Washington, A.E. (1993). Cost of ectopic pregnancy management: surgery versus methotrexate. *Fertility and Sterility*, **60**(6): 963–969.

DiMarchi, J.M., Cyka, R.E. (1992). Oral methotrexate for persistent ectopic pregnancy. A case report. *Journal of Reproductive Medicine*, **37**(7): 659–660.

DiMarchi, J.M., Kosasa, T.S., Kobara, T.Y., Hale, R.W. (1987). Persistent ectopic pregnancy. *Obstetrics and Gynecology*, **70**: 555–558.

Dumesic, D.A., Hafez, G.R. (1991). Delayed haemorrhage of a persistent ectopic pregnancy following laparoscopic salpingostomy and methotrexate therapy. *Obstetrics and Gynecology*, **78**: 960–962.

Eckford, S., Fox, R. (1993). Intratubal injection of prostaglandin in ectopic pregnancy. *Lancet*, **2**: 803.

Egarter, C., Husslein, P. (1988). Treatment of tubal pregnancy by prostaglandins. *Lancet*, **1**: 1104–1105.

Feichtinger, W., Kemeter, P. (1987). Conservative treatment of ectopic pregnancy by transvaginal aspiration under ultrasonographic control and methotrexate injection. *Lancet*, **1**: 381–382.

Feichtinger, W., Kemeter, P. (1989). Treatment of unruptured ectopic pregnancy by needling of sac and injection of methotrexate or PGE2 under transvaginal sonography control. *Archives of Gynecology and Obstetrics*, **246**: 85–89.

Fernandez, H., Baton, C., Lelaidier, C., Frydman, R. (1991). Conservative management of ectopic pregnancy: prospective randomised clinical trial of methotrexate versus prostaglandin sulprostone by combined transvaginal and systemic administration. *Fertility and Sterility*, **55**: 746–750.

Fernandez, H., Benifla, J.L., Lelaidier, C., Baton, C., Frydman, R. (1993). Methotrexate treatment of ectopic pregnancy: 100 cases treated by primary transvaginal injection under sonographic control. *Fertility and Sterility*, **59**(4): 773–777.

Fernandez, H., Rainhorn, J.D., Papiernik, E., Bellet, D., Frydman, R. (1988). Spontaneous resolution of ectopic pregnancy. *Obstetrics and Gynecology*, **71**: 171–174.

Fleischer, A.C., Kepple, D.M. (1992). *Transvaginal Sonography. A Clinical Atlas.* J B Lippincott, Philadelphia.

Frishman, G.N., Seifer, D.B. (1993). Hematosalpinx after methotrexate treatment of unruptured ectopic pregnancy. *Fertility and Sterility*, **60**(3): 571–572.

Glock, J.L., Johnson, J.V., Brumsted, J.R. (1994). Efficacy and safety of single-dose systemic methotrexate in the treatment of ectopic pregnancy. *Fertility and Sterility*, **62**(4): 716–721.

Groutz, A., Luxman, D., Cohen, J.R., David, M.P. (1993). Rising beta hCG titres following laparoscopic injection of methotrexate into unruptured, viable tubal pregnancies. *British Journal of Obstetrics and Gynaecology*, **100**: 286–287.

Higgins, K.A., Schwartz M.B. (1986). Treatment of persistent trophoblastic tissue after salpingostomy with methotrexate. *Fertility and Sterility*, **45**: 427–428.

Hoppe, D.E., Bekkar, B.E., Nager, C.W. (1994). Single-dose systemic methotrexate for the treatment of persistent ectopic pregnancy after conservative surgery. *Obstetrics and Gynecology*, **83**(1): 51–54.

Ichinoe, K., Wake, N., Shinkai, N., Shiina, Y., Miyazaki, Y., Tanaka, T. (1987). Non-surgical therapy to preserve oviduct function in patients with tubal pregnancies. *American Journal of Obstetrics and Gynecology*, **156**: 484–487.

Kenigsberg, D., Porte, J., Hull, M., Spitz, I.M. (1987). Medical treatment of residual ectopic pregnancy: RU486 and methotrexate. *Fertility and Sterility*, **47**: 702–703.

Kojima, E., Abe, Y., Morita, M., Ito, M., Hirakawa, S., Momose, K. (1990). The treatment of unruptured tubal pregnancy with intra-tubal methotrexate injection under laparoscopic control. *Obstetrics and Gynecology*, **75**: 723–725.

Kooi, S., Kock, H.C.L.V. (1990). Treatment of tubal pregnancy by local injection of methotrexate after adrenaline injection into the mesosalpinx: a report of 25 patients. *Fertility and Sterility*, **54**: 580–584.

Kooi, S., Kock, H.C.L.V. (1992). A review of the literature on the non-surgical treatment of tubal pregnancies. *Obstetrical and Gynecological Survey*, **47**: 739–749.

Lang, P.F., Weiss, P.A.M., Mayer, H.O. (1989). Local application of hyperosmolar glucose solution in tubal pregnancy. *Lancet*, **2**: 922–923.

Lang, P.F., Weiss, P.A.M., Mayer, H.O., Haas, J.G., Honigl, W. (1990). Conservative treatment of ectopic pregnancy with local injection of hyperosmolar glucose solution or prostaglandin F2. A prospective randomised study. *Lancet*, **2**: 78–81.

Lindblom, B. (1993). Non-surgical approaches in ectopic pregnancy: systemic medical treatment or local injection therapy. In: *Fallopian Tube: Advances in Diagnosis and Treatment*, (eds) T. Chard, J.G. Grudzinskas. Springer-Verlag, London. pp 271–277.

Lindblom, B., Hahlin, M., Kallfelt, B., Hamberger, L. (1987). Local prostaglandin F2 injection for termination of ectopic pregnancy. *Lancet*, **1**: 776–777.

Lindblom, B., Hahlin, M., Lundorff, P., Thorburn, J. (1990). Treatment of tubal pregnancy by laparoscopic-guided injection of prostaglandin PGF2 alpha. *Fertility and Sterility*, **54**: 404–408.

Lynch, L., Berkowitz, R.L., Chitkara, U., Alvarez, M. (1990). First trimester transabdominal multifetal pregnancy reduction: a report of 85 cases. *Obstetrics and Gynecology*, **75**: 735–738.

Menard, A., Crequat, J., Maldelbrot, L., Hanuy, J.P., Madelenat, P. (1991). Treatment of unruptured tubal pregnancy by local injection of methotrexate under transvaginal sonographic control. *Fertility and Sterility*, **54**: 47–50.

Mottla, G.L., Rulin, M.C., Guzick, D.S. (1992). Lack of resolution of ectopic pregnancy by intratubal injection of methotrexate. *Fertility and Sterility*, **57**(3): 685–687.

O'Shea, R.T., Thompson, G.R., Harding, A. (1994). Intra-amniotic methotrexate versus CO_2 laser laparoscopic salpingotomy in the management of tubal ectopic pregnancy – a prospective randomized trial. *Fertility and Sterility*, **62**(4): 876–878.

Ory, S.J., Nnadi, E., Herrmann, R., O'Brien, P.C., Melton, L.J. (1993). Fertility following ectopic pregnancy. *Fertility and Sterility*, **60**: 231–235.

Ory, S.J., Villanueva, A.L., Sand, P.K., Tamera, R.K. (1986). Conservative treatment of ectopic pregnancy with methotrexate. *American Journal of Obstetrics and Gynecology*, **154**: 1299–1306.

Pansky, M., Bukovsky, I., Golan, A., Herman, A., Hertziano, I., Langer, R., Caspi, E. (1992). Methotrexate local injection for unruptured tubal pregnancy: an alternative to laparotomy? *International Journal of Gynaecology and Obstetrics*, **37**(4): 265–270.

Paris, F.X., Henry-Suchet, J., Tesguier, L. (1986). The value of an anti-progesterone in the treatment of extrauterine pregnancy: Preliminary results. *Review Francais Gynecology et Obstetrique*, **81**: 607–609.

Parker, J., Thompson, D. (1994). Persistent ectopic pregnancy after conservative management successful treatment with single-dose intramuscular methotrexate. *Australia and New Zealand Journal of Obstetrics and Gynaecology*, **34**(1): 99–102.

Patsner, B., Keningsberg, D. (1988). Successful treatment of persistent ectopic pregnancy with oral methotrexate therapy. *Fertility and Sterility*, **50**: 982–983.

Pouly, J.L., Chapron, C., Manhes, H., Canis, M., Wattiez, A., Bruhat, M.A. (1991). Multifactorial analysis of fertility after conservative laparoscopic treatment of ectopic pregnancy in a series of 223 patients. *Fertility and Sterility*, **56**: 453–460.

Pouly, J.L., Mahnes, M., Mage, G., Canis, M., Bruhat, M.A. (1986). Conservative laparoscopic treatment of 321 ectopic pregnancies. *Fertility and Sterility*, **46**: 1093–1097.

Ransom, M.X., Garcia, A.J., Bohrer, M., Corsan, G.H., Kemmann, E. (1994). Serum progesterone as a predictor of methotrexate success in the treatment of ectopic pregnancy. *Obstetrics and Gynecology*, **83**(6): 1033–1037.

Risquez, F., Forman, R., Maleika, F., Foulot, H., Reidy, J., Chapman, M., Zorn, J.R. (1992a). Transcervical cannulation of the fallopian tube for the management of ectopic pregnancy: prospective multicenter study. *Fertility and Sterility*, **58**(6): 1131–1135.

Risquez, F., Mathieson, J., Zorn, J.R. (1990). Tubal cannulation via the cervix: a passing fancy or here to stay. *Journal of In Vitro Fertilization and Embryo Transfer*, **7**: 301–303.

Risquez, F., Pennehouat, G., Foulot, H., Mathieson, J., Dubuisson, J.B., Bonnin, A., Madelenat, P., Zorn, J.R. (1992b). Transcervical tubal cannulation and falloposcopy for the management of tubal pregnancy. *Human Reproduction*, **7**(2): 274–275.

Robertson, D.E., Hoye, M.A., Hansen, J.N. (1987). Reduction of ectopic pregnancy by injection under ultrasound control. *Lancet*, **2**: 974–975.

Rodi, I.A., Sauer, M.V., Gorill, M.J. (1986). The medical treatment of unruptured ectopic pregnancy with methotrexate and citrovorum rescue: preliminary experience. *Fertility and Sterility*, **46**: 811–813.

Russell, S.A., Filly, R.A., Damato, N. (1993). Sonographic diagnosis of ectopic pregnancy with endovaginal probes: what really has changed? *Journal of Ultrasound in Medicine*, **3**: 145–153.

Sauer, M.V., Greenberg, L.H., Gorrill, M.J. (1987). Non-surgical management of unruptured ectopic pregnancy: an extended clinical trial. *Fertility and Sterility*, **48**: 752–755.

Schoenfeld, A., Mashiah, R., Vardy, M., Ovadia, J. (1992). Methotrexate pneumonitis in non-surgical treatment of ectopic pregnancy. *Obstetrics and Gynecology*, **80**: 520–521.

Seifer, D.B., Gutmann, J.N., Grant, W.D., Kamps, C.A., DeCherney, A.H. (1993). Comparison of persistent ectopic pregnancy after laparoscopic salpingostomy versus salpingostomy at laparotomy for ectopic pregnancy. *Obstetrics and Gynecology*, **81**: 378–382.

Shapiro, B.S. (1987). The non-surgical management of ectopic pregnancy. *Clinical Obstetrics and Gynecology*, **30**: 230–235.

Stovall, T.G., Ling, F.W. (1993). Single dose methotrexate: an expanded clinical trial. *American Journal of Obstetrics and Gynecology*, **168**: 1759–1762.

Stovall, T.G., Ling, F.W., Gray, L.A. (1991a). Single dose methotrexate for treatment of ectopic pregnancy. *Obstetrics and Gynecology*, **77**: 754–757.

Stovall, T.G., Ling, F.W., Gray, L.A., Carson, S.A., Buster, J.E. (1991b). Methotrextae treatment of unruptured ectopic pregnancy: a report of 100 cases. *Obstetrics and Gynecology*, **77**: 749–753.

Tanaka, T., Hayashi, H., Kutsuzawa, T., Fujimoto, S., Ichinoe, K. (1982). Treatment of interstitial ectopic pregnancy with methotrexate: report of a successful case. *Fertility and Sterility*, **37**: 851–852.

Timor-Tritsch, I.E., Rottem, S. (1987). *Transvaginal sonography*. Elsevier, New York.

Timor-Tritsch, H., Baxi, L., Peisner, D.B. (1989). Transvaginal salpingocentesis: a new technique for treating ectopic pregnancy. *American Journal of Obstetrics and Gynecology*, **160**: 459–461.

Tulandi, T. (1992). Resolution and success of medical treatment of ectopic pregnancy. *Fertility and Sterility*, **57**(5): 963–964.

Tulandi, T., Hemmings, R., Khalifa, F. (1991). Rupture of ectopic pregnancy in women with low and declining serum beta chorionic gonadotropin concentration. *Fertility and Sterility*, **56**: 786–796.

Vermesh, M., Silva, P.D., Sauer, M.V., Vargyas, J.M., Lobo, R.A. (1988). Persistent tubal ectopic gestation: patterns of circulating beta human chorionic gonadotrophin and progesterone, and management options. *Fertility and Sterility*, **50**: 584–588.

Walden, P.A.M., Bagshawe, K.D. (1976). Reproductive performance of women successfully treated for gestational trophoblastic tumors. *American Journal of Obstetrics and Gynaecology*, **125**: 1108–1114.

Zakut, H., Sadan, O.O., Katz, A., Dreval, D., Bernstein, D. (1989). Management of tubal pregnancy with methotrexate. *British Journal of Obstetrics and Gynaecology*, **96**: 725–728.

CHAPTER 9

Conservative and expectant management of ectopic pregnancy

9.1 Introduction

In spite of the increased incidence of ectopic pregnancy in recent years the case fatality rate continues to fall. This may result from the widespread introduction of diagnostic tests and an increasing awareness by patients and their doctors of the serious nature of this disease. Consequently, the rate of tubal rupture (and hence dramatic presentation with life-threatening symptoms and signs) has become as low as 20% (Pansky et al., 1991). Whether this trend will be seen in other parts of the world remains uncertain. What is clear is the increasing need for conservative and/or expectant forms of management to deal with that large group of women who present early with subacute ectopic pregnancy, i.e. our patients in group 3 (Balasch and Barri, 1994). For the purposes of this chapter, expectant management is defined as non-medical and non-surgical management and conservative treatment is any surgical operation in which the tube is conserved. Except where specifically stated, the management of a first ectopic pregnancy is discussed.

9.2 The choices

The treatment of ectopic pregnancy entails numerous choices by the physician: (i) whether to attempt it (expectant versus surgical or medical treatment); (ii) choice of route (laparoscopy, laparotomy, sonographic or transcervical); (iii) choice of operation (conservative versus radical); and (iv) choice of surgical approach (standard techniques versus micro-surgery). The ideal management in an individual case depends on a number of variables, the principal ones being the location and size of the ectopic pregnancy and whether the tube has ruptured (Figure 9.1). Other deciding factors include the anatomical status of the pelvis and particularly the

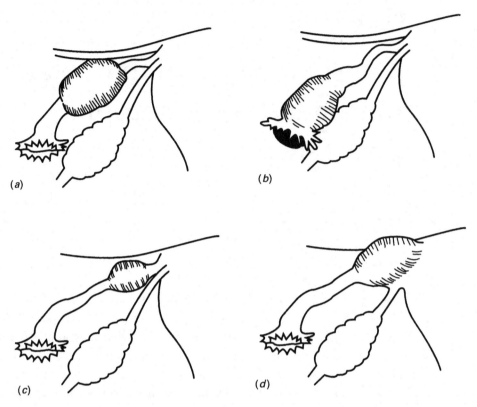

Figure 9.1 Ectopic pregnancy located in (*a*) ampullary, (*b*) infundibular, (*c*) isthmic and (*d*) cornual portion of the fallopian tube.

health of the unaffected tube, the availability of microsurgical techniques and the wishes of the patient. Past surgical and obstetrical history is also relevant. Whatever the chosen form of treatment, diagnostic laparoscopy is central to the management strategy: it allows the diagnosis to be confirmed in almost all cases, the state of the pelvis to be determined and opens the possibility of laparoscopic treatment.

9.3   Expectant management

There is now considerable evidence that some ectopic pregnancies can spontaneously abort in the same manner as intrauterine pregnancies (Ohel *et al.*, 1980; Garcia *et al.*, 1987; Sauer *et al.*, 1987; Fernandez *et al.*, 1988; Atri *et al.*, 1993). The basis of expectant management is that a significant percentage of ectopic pregnancies are diagnosed at a very early stage (at least in the western world), some of which would be expected to resolve spontaneously (Cox and Steinberg, 1942; Lund, 1955). This so called spontaneous 'cure' is said to have occurred in 'mild' cases of ectopic pregnancy, most of which remain undiagnosed because surgical intervention is not performed. Previously these could only be conclusively diagnosed if subsequent histology of the tube demonstrated the presence of old hyalinised villi (Burrows *et al.*, 1980). Spontaneous regression of an ectopic pregnancy has also been described as a 'missed tubal abortion', with analogy to intrauterine events. Although certainly more common than previously thought, the incidence of spontaneous regression depends entirely on how carefully one looks for it. In one study, 7% of tubal pregnancies presented with human chorionic gonadotrophin (hCG) levels of less than 50 IU/L, and in approximately half of these women, fibrotic degenerating chorionic tissue was noted on light microscopic examination of the fallopian tube. These three patients presented with hCG values of less than 13 IU/L (Thorburn *et al.*, 1983). Another mechanism put forward for the unexpected finding of spontaneous resolution of an ectopic pregnancy is that of a 'complete tubal abortion', again by analogy with spontaneous complete abortion. This abortion is often asymptomatic or may present with minor vaginal bleeding or transient abdominal pain. One such case was reported by Ohel and colleagues (1980) who studied a tubal pregnancy conception cycle in a previously infertile woman. This particular patient was asymptomatic and recovered without medical or surgical treatment. It is not known how often this occurs.

Lund (1955) reported a comparative study of two similar groups of patients with ectopic pregnancy who were considered stable and in whom immediate surgery was not essential. The diagnosis of ectopic pregnancy was on the basis of a positive qualitative urinary pregnancy test (Aschheim-Zondek or Friedman test) and curettage. It is certainly possible that at least some of these patients did not actually have an ectopic pregnancy. Fifty-seven percent of 119 patients managed expectantly were considered 'cured'. Surgery was required in the remaining cases, sometimes up to four weeks after admission, primarily for the presence of persistent trophoblast. There was no difference in the subsequent intrauterine pregnancy rate (45%) between the two groups; neither was the rate of repeat ectopic pregnancy (15%) increased in the group managed expectantly. As might be expected, however, the women treated surgically returned home considerably sooner. This may have been the reason why this non-surgical approach fell into disrepute. More recent reports of an 80% spontaneous resolution rate of laparoscopically-confirmed ectopic pregnancy, has regenerated interest in this form of 'non-treatment' (Mashiach *et al.*, 1982; Carp *et al.*, 1986; Derricks *et al.*, 1987; Garcia *et al.*, 1987; Sauer *et al.*, 1987; Fernandez *et al.*, 1988; Makinen *et al.*, 1990;

Atri *et al.*, 1993). The precise criteria for entry into these studies varied. In all cases, the patients were clinically stable with no evidence of tubal rupture. In some studies, patients were included if there was no bleeding from the fimbrial end of the tube whereas others considered distension of the tube overlying the pregnancy as a contraindication to expectant management. In the majority of studies reported to date, the size of the resolving ectopic pregnancies as measured by transvaginal sonography (TVS) ranged from 1 cm to 3.5 cm and the serum beta hCG levels were typically less than 1000 IU/L (Fernandez *et al.*, 1988; Makinen *et al.*, 1990; Atri *et al.*, 1993). These authors concluded that the more advanced, vascular ectopic pregnancies with higher hCG levels are less likely to resolve spontaneously. In one study, however, one-third of ectopic pregnancies that resolved spontaneously initially enlarged and developed mild vascularity with increased pelvic fluid at follow-up TVS. These findings, therefore, should not, in and of themselves, indicate failure of 'treatment', provided serum beta hCG levels continue to fall and the patient remains stable (Atri *et al.*, 1993). On the basis of the small studies cited above, nine of the 20 patients successfully managed expectantly who were desirous of pregnancy and were known to have patent tubes on hysterosalpingography (HSG) subsequently gave birth (Carp *et al.*, 1986; Garcia *et al.*, 1987; Fernandez *et al.*, 1988; Atri *et al.*, 1993). There were also four spontaneous abortions and one repeat ectopic in this group. Clearly, these numbers are too small to determine whether the long-term reproductive outcome of expectant management is any better than that of other forms of treatment.

In their recent review, Pansky *et al.* (1991) reported on a meta-analysis of 61 patients who were treated expectantly. They concluded that the role for this form of non-invasive 'treatment' is limited to that subgroup of patients who are minimally symptomatic and in whom serum hCG levels are falling. Ylostalo *et al.* (1992) estimate this group to be 25% of all women with an ectopic pregnancy diagnosed before six weeks' gestation. They have suggested that if emergency surgery is not needed, serum hCG estimation and TVS be repeated at intervals of one to two days. If the hCG level is falling, then expectant management can be used with caution, because there has been one case report of a tubal rupture following decline of beta hCG from 5620 IU/L to 960 IU/L (Gretz and Quagliarello, 1987). If the hCG level starts to increase or clinical symptoms and sonographic findings become suspicious, then active management is recommended. Others would include the observation that the gestational sac is not increasing in size and the patient is thought to be a high risk surgical candidate (Zacur, 1993).

There are potential disadvantages to the expectant management of laparoscopically-diagnosed ectopic pregnancy. For example, in-traperitoneal bleeding may not be completely reabsorbed and there may be continued peritoneal irritation and subsequently adhesion formation when the tubal abortion is managed conservatively. Rarely, dense pelvic adhesions may wall off the ectopic pregnancy, the so-called 'chronic ectopic' (Cole and Corlett, 1982). [This term is also used when a tubal, usually isthmic, pregnancy ruptures into the broad ligament. A haema-toma may form, which may be asymptomatic for several weeks. As the pregnancy grows, the broad ligament itself may rupture, and rarely a secondary abdominal pregnancy develops.] The consequences of pelvic adhesions include tubal occlusion with subsequent infertility and, rarely, secondary abdominal pregnancy. According to this hypothesis, these seri-ous long-term complications of expectant management of an ectopic pregnancy are related to the degree of intraperitoneal bleeding associated with the pregnancy. This would explain why some early ectopic pregnan-cies resolve completely whereas others persist for a few weeks. Limited information provided by HSG and repeat laparoscopy in patients managed with this non-intervention policy, do not support the view that chronic trophoblast proliferation and tubal damage are likely (Garcia *et al.*, 1987). However there are other disadvantages of expectant management includ-ing the need for emergency laparotomy, the financial cost of serial hCG measurements and TVS procedures and the emotional cost from the anxiety of waiting for several days (up to 45 days in one study) to deter-mine whether the 'treatment' has been successful (Zacur, 1993).

At present it is not possible to recommend routine expectant manage-ment in the small unruptured tubal pregnancy, primarily because ran-domised controlled trials comparing conservative (usually laparoscopic) surgery and expectant management are not available. Such a study will be ethically difficult because laparoscopic confirmation of the diagnosis is essential, whether or not laparoscopic surgery is then performed. This will mean that some women may have to undergo two separate procedures, if expectant management should fail. Based solely on case reports, there is no particular advantage to the non-surgical approach in terms of future fertility, whereas prolonged hospitalisation in such women is a distinct disadvantage.

9.4   Surgical management: laparoscopy, laparotomy or both?

Surgical approaches that conserve the fallopian tube are performed in only 12% of cases treated in the USA even though they have been available for several decades (Young *et al.*, 1991).

The evidence in favour of laparoscopic diagnosis and treatment of ectopic pregnancy is overwhelming. Laparoscopic surgery can be used in the treatment of most cases of ectopic pregnancy, both ruptured and unruptured (Silva, 1988). The principal advantage is that diagnosis and treatment are effected by a single procedure. Other advantages include shorter hospitalisation time (Zouves *et al.*, 1992), faster return to domestic activities and work (Brumsted *et al.*, 1988) and 50% reduction in overall costs (Baumann *et al.*, 1991) compared with laparotomy. Outcomes in terms of pregnancy rates and adhesion formation following laparoscopic surgery are at least as good as after laparotomy (Vermesh *et al.*, 1989; Lundorff *et al.*, 1991b). If laparotomy is to be used, magnification and fibreoptic headlamps (microsurgery) are extremely useful.

The major contraindications to laparoscopic treatment of an ectopic pregnancy are massive intra-abdominal bleeding with clinical shock and extensive intra-abdominal adhesions (Zouves *et al.*, 1992). Laparoscopic procedures can be performed on ectopic pregnancies which are ruptured or leaking, even up to 10 cm in diameter (Baumann *et al.*, 1991; Koninckx *et al.*, 1991), provided that vital signs are stable.

9.4.1   THE TECHNIQUE

Laparoscopy is performed in the usual manner (Section 5.4); the details are well described in the literature (Semm, 1979; Gomel *et al.*, 1986), to which the interested reader is encouraged to refer. Briefly, the procedure can be performed using a double or triple puncture technique: the subumbilical incision for the laparoscope, and either one or two additional access channels for insertion of a grasping and operating instrument. Manipulation of the uterus via a uterine cannula facilitates the intervention, and particularly exposure, of the affected tube. This is contraindicated if a co-existing intrauterine pregnancy is suspected. The procedure is usually performed in the modified Trendelenburg position. If available, the gynaecologist might perform the procedure by viewing a television monitor (videopelviscopy) (Magos *et al.*, 1988 and 1989).

At exploratory laparoscopy the surgeon determines the exact location of the pregnancy (typically revealed as a bulge in the tube), the condition of the involved tube, that of the opposite tube and ovary and the importance of any existing pelvic abnormalities. Occasionally, it is impossible to be certain of the presence of a tubal pregnancy, in which case, the whole pelvis and bowel should be systematically inspected to exclude rare cases of extratubal pregnancy. What should the operator do if despite the strong clinical suspicion of an ectopic pregnancy, laparoscopy is negative? This may occur in very early ectopic pregnancy (Yaffe *et al.*, 1979) or when distorted tubal anatomy precludes a good view of the pelvis. There are two schools of thought here. The first (the hawks) would proceed to laparotomy, on the assumption that the patient's clinical condition warrants exclusion of the diagnosis. This is probably justified when adhesions impair the view, as half these patients have an ectopic pregnancy (Esposito, 1980). On the other hand, the doves would keep a close eye on the patient with serial ultrasound and beta hCG measurements. Should symptoms, signs, ultrasound abnormalities or the beta hCG levels fail to regress, most would repeat the laparoscopy, and then proceed to laparotomy. The disadvantage of this wait-and-see approach is that the patient undergoes two anaesthetics; on the other hand an unnecessary laparotomy may be avoided.

Various methods are available to open the tube, such as electrocautery (unipolar or bipolar), laser (argon, or CO_2) or surgical instruments (Johns and Hardy, 1984; Thornton *et al.*, 1991). Choosing between them is more a matter of preference and availability rather than a real difference in performance. Once the tube has been opened, the trophoblast is removed and suction/irrigation used for evacuation. The most difficult aspect of any laparoscopic procedure is the occasional inability to achieve complete haemostasis at the site of placental attachment on the interior tubal wall, from the cut edges of the salpingostomy incision or from trauma to the fimbriae. Apart from the standard methods of securing haemostasis such as digital pressure on the tube, meticulous electrocoagulation of the bleeding points, injection of an oxytocic into the tubal wall and ligation of the mesosalpingeal vessels, ingenious methods have been devised to manage this problem. These include inserting a Foley catheter through the fimbrial end of the tube to reach the bleeding site and then distending it for up to 12 hours post-operatively. The Foley can be removed through a separate abdominal incision (Fuchs, 1982). If haemostasis cannot be achieved then laparotomy is essential.

Surgery on the opposite tube noted to be damaged at the time of conservative surgery is probably best delayed to take advantage of carefully controlled conditions such as surgical experience and the availability of microsurgical tools. Some would recommend an adhesion prevention regimen after removal of the tubal pregnancy. The pelvis is first filled with heparinised (5000 U/L) Ringer's lactate; blood and debris are removed by aspiration. This is followed by instillation of 32% Dextran 70. The efficacy of this and other similar techniques is uncertain.

9.4.2   COMBINED LAPAROSCOPY AND MINILAPAROTOMY

Minimally invasive surgery in the management of gynaecological emergencies is believed by some to have physiological, psychological, economic and cosmetic advantages (Magos *et al.*, 1989). Others have suggested that combined laparoscopy and mini-laparotomy (or extracorporeal laparoscopic technique) be considered as an alternative to the technically more complex procedure of videopelviscopy (Loffer, 1986; Taylor and Cumming, 1979; Johnson, 1993). The procedure involves exteriorising the fallopian tube through a 2 cm suprapubic incision, after confirming the diagnosis by laparoscopy. Salpingectomy was successfully performed using this technique in ten of 12 patients with isthmic or ampullary ectopic pregnancy, although in three cases it was necessary to re-establish a pneumoperitoneum (Johnson, 1993). Laparotomy may be necessary if the tube tears. In any case, the procedure ends with a final re-examination of the abdomen to confirm that haemostasis is secure and that the tube is not stuck to the anterior abdominal wall. It has been suggested that the tube should be exteriorised under laparoscopic vision whenever a distally sited ectopic pregnancy needs to be excised from a mobile tube in a thin patient. This is particularly suitable in those units lacking the sophisticated equipment of video laparoscopy or the availability of adequately trained gynaecological endoscopists. Inpatient stay is shortened by three days (Taylor and Cumming, 1979).

9.4.3   COMPLICATIONS

Apart from vascular, bowel and urinary tract injury, the complications of laparoscopic treatment of an ectopic pregnancy include persistent trophoblast (Section 8.2.3) and delayed bleeding. Incomplete removal of trophoblast was reported in 15 of 321 patients treated by laparoscopy (Pouly *et al.*, 1986). Half of them required a second laparoscopy; the remainder underwent salpingostomy by laparotomy. The alternative is to use medical treatment in this situation (Chapter 8). At least in the USA, most patients undergoing treatment for ectopic pregnancy, whether medical, surgical or expectant, are followed up with serial serum hCG measurements in an attempt to detect any persistent trophoblast. The long-term effect of this complication on tubal function is unknown. By contrast, delayed bleeding is rare, but potentially fatal. Close monitoring in a hospital setting for at least 12–24 hours is recommended by most gynaecologists.

9.5   Surgical management: choice of operation

Surgery remains the treatment of choice for most patients with an ectopic pregnancy, but the trend is moving away from open salpingectomy. The indications for this and other radical procedures are considered in Chapter 10. Conservativism should not be confused with complacency (Saunders, 1990). The major advantage of conservative surgery is that it preserves future fertility (DeCherney *et al.*, 1981, 1982). Therefore, a conservative procedure should perhaps be considered the first line of surgical treatment for all ectopic pregnancies whether ruptured or not. Should uncontrollable bleeding follow, a more radical procedure, e.g. salpingectomy, may be carried out. We shall describe here the choice of conservative operation in relation to the site of an ectopic pregnancy. In each case the aim of the procedure is to remove the ectopic pregnancy with minimal injury to the tube, resulting in a balance between the incidence of subsequent intrauterine pregnancy and repeat ectopic pregnancy (Gomel, 1983).

The surgical choice in the unruptured fimbrial pregnancy lies between a salpingotomy-type procedure performed either by laparoscopy or by microsurgical laparotomy and fimbrial evacuation. Some would argue that the same choice applies to the mid-tubal ampullary pregnancy (the most common form of tubal ectopic pregnancy), but others would not consider fimbrial evacuation suitable in this case. Each will be considered in turn.

9.5.1   LINEAR SALPINGOTOMY

Linear salpingotomy is the term used to describe a linear incision on the anti-mesenteric border of the tube over the ectopic pregnancy (Figure 9.2). A number of techniques can be used to open the tube: (i) coagulation and/or cutting diathermy (cautery); (ii) surgical knife; and (iii) laser (CO_2, argon or Nd:Yag). Most units will use a combination of the first and second. The main advantage of laser surgery is its precision.

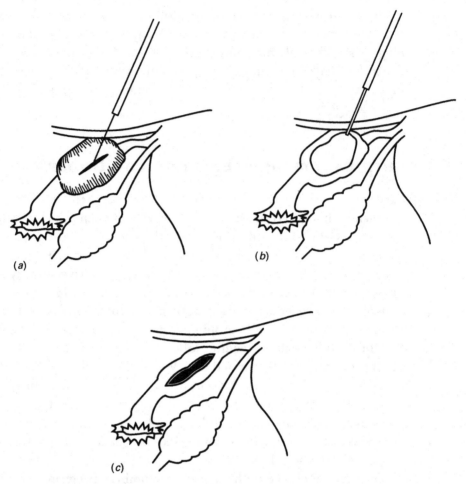

Figure 9.2 Linear salpingostomy. A linear incision is performed on the anti-mesenteric border of the fallopian tube and the products of conception are removed. The evacuated tube is left to heal.

The depth of destruction is easily controlled (thermal effect of up to 500 1 μm in CO_2 laser), hence allowing atruamatic tissue incision. It has been suggested that the CO_2 laser is perhaps the least appropriate tool for this purpose, because although it is less likely to damage tubal tissues by virtue of its minimal depth of tissue penetration, the effect on the tissues is vaporising rather than haemostatic. One would therefore expect blood loss to be greater with the CO_2 laser, although this has not be confirmed in two small studies (Paulson and Asmar, 1989; Koninckx *et al.*, 1991). Others have suggested that when adhesions limit mobilisation of the tube, rapid adhesiolysis is better effected by means of the CO_2 laser than electrosurgery (Koninckx *et al.*, 1991). Despite the theoretical advantages of laser surgery, there are, as yet, no randomised controlled studies comparing its use with that of electrocautery in laparoscopic treatment of tubal pregnancy. Pregnancy rates after these procedures are discussed in Chapter 11.

The length of the incision is a matter of judgement. It should be just long enough to allow the products of conception to be removed with ease. This is usually performed using grasping forceps in a piecemeal fashion until only necrotic material is left at the site of implantation. Most would not advocate removing this necrotic material as extensive haemorrhage often follows. There is approximately a 4% risk of a persistent trophoblast (Pouly *et al.*, 1986).

Reducing bleeding from the operative site is principally a matter of personal choice (for options see Section 9.4.1). The injection of a dilute pitressin solution (1–2 ml of 10 IU diluted in 100 ml) along the incision is advocated by some to minimise blood loss. Perhaps the only theoretical disadvantage of this approach is that an oxytocic might delay significant bleeding to when the operation is over.

Once the products of conception have been removed and the bleeding points secured, the next decision centres on whether to close the linear salpingotomy incision. When left open, the term salpingostomy is used (DeCherney *et al.*, 1982). The arguments in favour of closing the tube include haemostasis and attempting to minimise post-operative adhesions by eliminating all raw surfaces within the pelvis. Others would argue that tissue ischaemia and consequently adhesion formation may be induced by wound closure. As the conceptus does not usually lie within the tubal lumen, a correctly performed linear salpingotomy should not extend into the cavity of the fallopian tube and therefore, at least theoretically, closure of the incision is unecessary to maintain tubal patency. If the tube is to be closed, interrupted 6-0 or 8-0 synthetic absorbable sutures are used.

9.5.2   FIMBRIAL EVACUATION

Fimbrial evacuation or milking out of the tube is the alternative to linear salpingotomy when the pregnancy lies in the fimbrial region (Langer *et al.*, 1987). This is performed at open laparotomy by holding and compressing the tube gently, starting just proximal to the site of the pregnancy and moving systematically to the fimbrial end of the tube. The whole procedure should be performed with great care and in the gentlest fashion. The alternative is to remove the distal pregnancy through the tubal ostium at laparoscopy by so-called tubal aspiration (Bruhat *et al.*,

1980). Most would only do this when a tubal abortion is in progress and the tubal contents are seen to protrude through the distal tubal opening.

Despite the theoretical advantages of minimal surgical intervention, milking out the tube remains a controversial procedure, especially when performed for the treatment of an ampullary rather than a fimbrial pregnancy. Although it is easy to perform, this approach may be associated with complications such as tubal damage (e.g. a false passage) with subsequent scarring and adhesion formation, continued bleeding from the implantation site and persistent trophoblast (Brosens *et al.*, 1984). The histopathology of the developing tubal pregnancy suggests that in a large proportion of cases extraluminal spread of trophoblast takes place (Budowick *et al.*, 1980). The fact that most of the conceptus lies between the tube and the peritoneum militates against the deceptively simple process of milking out the tube. This may also account for the approximately 4% risk of persistent trophoblast tissue remaining after conservative surgery (a figure that is remarkably similar for all forms of non-radical surgery). Typically there is a latency of one to four weeks before symptoms re-appear; therefore, serial hCG measurements are recommended until non-pregnant levels are reached (Lundorff *et al.*, 1991a).

It has been suggested that if fimbrial evacuation is to be attempted, only gentle pressure should be applied, and if complete expression of the products of conception cannot be achieved, then linear salpingotomy should be performed. The reasoning behind this is that an intact, viable pregnancy (whether fimbrial or ampullary) is likely to be firmly adherent to the tubal subserosa; it is very unlikely that this can be successfully milked out. If the pregnancy is non-viable it is probably less firmly attached to the tubal wall and fimbrial evacuation is more likely to succeed. It has been suggested that the less viable ectopic (with marked necrosis of chorionic tissue and which is poorly attached to the tubal wall) might present with lower hCG levels, and hence could be identified prior to surgery as being suitable for fimbrial evacuation (Sherman *et al.*, 1987).

Clearly, this procedure is only appropriate for distal tubal gestations that are loosely adherent within the tubal lumen; these are usually expressed with minimal effort. If anything more than very minor tubal pressure does not effect evacuation of the tube, the procedure should be abandoned. The rate of intrauterine pregnancy is reportedly lower and that of repeat ectopic pregnancy is higher after this procedure in comparison to other forms of surgical treatment (Timonen and Niemenen, 1967), but more recent studies by proponents of the technique have given better results (Langer *et al.*, 1987; Sherman *et al.*, 1987). More details are given in Chapter 11.

9.5.3   MID-TUBAL RESECTION

When confronted with a mid-tubal ectopic pregnancy three surgical procedures are available to the surgeon. The first, linear salpingotomy is useful when the tube is intact; this can be performed either by laparoscopy or through microsurgical laparotomy. The second procedure, mid-tubal resection with or without end-to-end anastomosis, is necessary when the tube has ruptured or control of bleeding is felt to be inadequate. The third option is milking the tube, but for reasons stated above, most have abandoned this procedure unless the pregnancy lies at the fimbrial portion of the tube.

9.5.3.1   *The Technique*

Mid-tubal resection is best performed using magnification provided by ocular loupes or the operating microscope as described by Winston and Margara (1980) and Patton and Kistner (1984) among others. The first step is to excise the tubal segment. This is followed by atraumatically removing blood clots from both tubal segments, irrigation and haemostasis. If magnification is not available, the tubal segments are ligated with 4-0 synthetic absorbable material, preserving as much of the tubal length as possible, until such time as microsurgical re-anastomosis can be performed (DeCherney *et al.*, 1980). Re-anastomosis is usually ampullary to isthmic using either single or double layer closure with 6-0 or 8-0 suture. Some have recommended transfundal lavage using the Buxton clamp or by passing a blunt probe through the fimbrial end across the line of anastomosis (Patton and Kistner, 1984).

9.5.4   ISTHMIC TUBAL PREGNANCY

Unlike the ampullary ectopic, the isthmic tubal pregnancy usually extends into the lumen of the fallopian tube. Furthermore, its proximity to the cornual region of the uterus makes bleeding more of a problem at this site. Hence, resection of the tubal segment or partial salpingectomy is the preferred treatment in these cases. Uterotubal implantation and cornual resection of the intramural tube are no longer performed.

9.5.5   REPEAT ECTOPIC PREGNANCY

At least one in five or six women with one ectopic pregnancy will develop another. The best management of those unfortunate women who develop a second pregnancy in the same tube previously treated conservatively is uncertain (Oelsner, 1987). In spite of favourable case reports (DeCherney *et al.*, 1985), it is logical that the repeat ectopic pregnancy rate should be much higher after two ectopics in the same tube than after only one. Some would therefore recommend a radical procedure (such as salpingectomy) in this situation. As *in-vitro* fertilisation–embryo transfer (IVF-ET), which has a take-home-baby-rate of approximately 10%, remains the only hope for future pregnancies in women lacking any fallopian tube, the option of performing another conservative procedure becomes more attractive. Moreover, the live birth rate after salpingostomy in the sole remaining tube is approximately 40% with a repeat ectopic pregnancy rate of 20%. The choice is a difficult one and clearly all options need to be discussed with the couple prior to surgery. The woman with no living children may opt for another conservative procedure, in the hope of a viable pregnancy, whereas her sister may prefer to avoid the trauma of another ectopic pregnancy and prefer the option of a radical procedure. The choice is theirs.

9.6   Management of heterotopic pregnancy

Heterotopic pregnancy, the combination of intrauterine and extrauterine pregnancy, deserves particular attention. Once thought to be extremely rare, its incidence in spontaneous conceptions is now believed to range between one in 4000 and one in 7000 pregnancies and is even higher (1–3% of all clinical pregnancies) after IVF-ET. Nevertheless, heterotopic pregnancy remains a difficult diagnostic (Section 1.7) and management problem.

Patients still present with haemorrhagic shock (Lund *et al.*, 1989). Delay in diagnosis is commonly the result of symptoms being attributed to the complications of intrauterine pregnancy. hCG levels are often in the normal range in a heterotopic pregnancy; therefore, early diagnosis depends on maintaining a high index of suspicion, particularly following gamete manipulation, pelvic surgery or a history of pelvic inflammatory disease. The earlier the diagnosis is made, the more likely it is that a conservative therapeutic approach will be successful in improving the prognosis of the intrauterine pregnancy while keeping maternal mortality and morbidity to a minimium.

Although the diagnosis is being made earlier by TVS (Rein *et al.*,1989; Guirgis and Craft, 1991; Fa and Gerscovich, 1993), laparoscopy is often helpful. This should be followed by the least invasive therapeutic regimen available to ensure continuing viability of the intrauterine pregnancy. Treatment with mifepristone and potassium chloride has been reported with varying degrees of success (Levin *et al.*, 1990; Fernandez *et al.*, 1993). In most cases, simple removal of the ectopic pregnancy while avoiding intrauterine instrumentation will suffice. In the absence of any evidence of abortion, three quarters of the intrauterine pregnancies go to term (Sondheimer *et al.*, 1985; Yovich *et al.*, 1985; Bearman *et al.*, 1986; Porter *et al.*, 1986; ; McLain and Kirkwood, 1987; Bassil *et al.*, 1991; Goldman *et al.*, 1991).

9.7 Point summary

1. Expectant management: if emergency surgery is not needed, serum hCG estimation and TVS are repeated at intervals of one to two days. Active management is recommended if the hCG level rises or suspicious clinical symptoms and sonographic findings develop.

2. Potential disadvantages of expectant management include continued peritoneal irritation and subsequently adhesion formation, tubal occlusion, infertility and rarely, secondary abdominal pregnancy.

3. There is no particular advantage to the expectant approach in terms of future fertility, whereas prolonged hospitalisation in such women is a distinct disadvantage.

4. Laparoscopic surgery can be used to both diagnose and treat most cases of both ruptured and unruptured ectopic pregnancy, provided vital signs are stable. The major contraindications are massive intra-abdominal bleeding and extensive intra-abdominal adhesions.

5. Laparoscopic treatment of tubal pregnancy offers numerous advantages: reduced operating time, hospital stay and cost, earlier return to activity and improved cosmetic result.

6. Linear salpingotomy is the most widely used procedure when the tube is intact. The term salpingostomy is used when the tube is left open to heal by secondary intention.

7. Fertility rates after salpingotomy via laparoscopy or laparotomy are comparable.

8. Fimbrial evacuation should only be performed if the pregnancy is already aborting through the tube; it should be abandonded if anything more than very minor tubal pressure does not effect evacuation of the distal pregnancy.

9. Mid-tubal resection with or without end to end anastomosis is necessary when the tube has ruptured or bleeding control is inadequate.

10. Most cases of heterotopic pregnancy are managed by simple removal of the ectopic while avoiding intrauterine instrumentation. In the absence of any evidence of abortion, three-quarters of the intrauterine pregnancies go to term.

9.8   References

Atrash, H.K., MacKay, H.T., Hogue, C.J.R. (1990). Ectopic pregnancy concurrent with induced abortion: incidence and mortality. *American Journal of Obstetrics and Gynecology*, **162**: 726–730.

Atri, M., Bret, P.M., Tulandi, T. (1993). Spontaneous resolution of ectopic pregnancy: initial appearance and evolution at transvaginal ultrasound. *Radiology*, **186**: 83–86.

Balasch, J., Barri, P. (1994). Treatment of ectopic pregnancy: the new gynaecological dilemma. *Human Reproduction*, **9**: 547–558.

Bassil, S., Pouly, J.L., Canis, M., Janny, L., Vye, P., Chapron, C., Bruhat, M.A. (1991). Advanced heterotopic pregnancy after *in-vitro* fertilization and embryo transfer, with survival of both the babies and the mother. *Human Reproduction*, **6**(7):1008–1010.

Baumann, R., Magos, A.L., Turnbull, A. (1991). Prospective comparison of videopelviscopy with laparotomy for ectopic pregnancy. *British Journal of Obstetrics and Gynaecology*, **98**: 765–771.

Bearman, D.M., Vieta, P.A., Snipes, R.D. (1986). Heterotopic pregnancy after *in vitro* fertilization and embryo transfer. *Fertility and Sterility*, **45**: 719–721.

Brosens, I., Gordts, S., Vasquez, G., Boeckx, W. (1984). Function retaining surgical management of ectopic pregnancy. *European Journal of Obstetrics Gynaecology Reproductive Biology*, **18**: 395–402.

Bruhat, M.A., Manhes, H, Mage, G. (1980). Treatment of ectopic pregnancy by means of laparoscopy. *Fertility and Sterility*, **33**: 411–414.

Brumsted, J., Kessler, C., Gibson, C., Nakajima, S., Riddick, D.H., Gibson, M. (1988). A comparison of laparoscopy and laparotomy for the treatment of ectopic pregnancy. *Obstetrics and Gynaecology*, **71**: 889–892.

Budowick, M., Johnson, T.R.B., Genadry, R., Parmley, T.H., Woodruff, J.D. (1980). The histopathology of the developing tubal ectopic pregnancy. *Fertility and Sterility*, **34**: 169–171.

Burrows, S., Moors, W., Pekala, B. (1980). Missed tubal abortion. *American Journal of Obstetrics and Gynecology*, **136**: 691–692.

Carp, H.J., Oelsner, G., Serr, D.M., Mashiah, S. (1986). Fertility after non-surgical treatment of ectopic pregnancy. *Journal of Reproductive Medicine*, **31**: 119–122.

Cole, T., Corlett, R.C. Jr. (1982). Chronic ectopic pregnancy. *Obstetrics and Gynecology*, **59**: 63–88.

Cox, M.E., Steinberg, M. (1942). Bilateral tubal pregnancy. *American Journal of Obstetrics and Gynecology*, **43**: 120–123.

DeCherney, A.H., Maheaux, R., Naftolin, F. (1982). Salpingostomy for ectopic pregnancy in the sole patent oviduct: reproductive outcome. *Fertility and Sterility*, **37**: 619–622.

DeCherney, A.H., Polan, M.L., Kort, H., Kase, N. (1980). Microsurgical technique in the management of tubal ectopic pregnancy. *Fertility and Sterility*, **34**: 324–327.

DeCherney, A.H., Romero, R., Naftolin, F. (1981). Surgical management of unruptured ectopic pregnancy. *Fertility and Sterility*, **35**: 21–24.

DeCherney, A.H., Silidker, J.S., Mezer, H.C., Tarlatzis, B.C. (1985). Reproductive outcome following two ectopic pregnancies. *Fertility and Sterility*, **43**: 82–89.

Derricks, T., Scholz, C., Tauber, H. (1987). Spontaneous recovery of ectopic pregnancy: a preliminary report. *European Journal of Obstetrics, Gynecology and Reproductive Biology*, **25**: 181–185.

Esposito, V.M. (1980). Ectopic pregnancy: the laparoscope as a diagnostic aid. *Journal of Reproductive Medicine*, **25**: 17–23.

Fa, E.M., Gerscovich, E.O. (1993). High resolution ultrasound in the diagnosis of heterotopic pregnancy: combined transabdominal and transvaginal approach. *British Journal of Obstetrics and Gynaecology*, **100**(9): 871–2.

Fernandez, H., Lelaidier, C., Doumerc, S., Fournet, P., Olivennes, F., Frydman, R. (1993). Non-surgical treatment of heterotopic pregnancy: a report of six cases. *Fertility and Sterility*, **60**(3): 428–432.

Fernandez, H., Rainhorn, J., Papiernick, E., Bellet, D., Frydman, R. (1988). Spontaneous resolution of ectopic pregnancy. *Obstetrics and Gynecology*, **71**: 171–174.

Franklin, E.W., Zeiderman, A.M., Lammele, P. (1973). Tubal ectopic pregnancy: etiology, obstetric and gynecologic sequelae. *American Journal of Obstetrics and Gynaecology*, **117**: 220–225.

Fuchs, T. (1982). Conservative operative treatment of ectopic pregnancy. *Acta Obstetrica Gynecologica Scandinavica*, **61**: 519–525.

Garcia, A., Aubert, J., Sama, J., Josimovich, J. (1987). Expectant management of presumed ectopic pregnancy. *Fertility and Sterility*, **48**: 395–400.

Goldman, J.A., Dicker, D., Dekel, A., Feldberg, D., Ashkenazi, J.

(1991). Successful management and outcome of heterotopic triplet *in-vitro* fertilization (IVF) gestation: twin tubal and surviving intrauterine pregnancy. *Journal of In-Vitro Fertilization and Embryo Transfer*, **8**(5): 300–302.

Gomel, V. (1983). *Microsurgery in Female Infertility*. Little Brown and Company, Boston.

Gomel, V., Taylor, P.J., Yuzpe, A.A., Rioux, J. (1986). *Laparoscopy and Hysteroscopy in Gynecologic Practice*. Year Book Medical Publishers, Chicago.

Gretz, G., Quagliarello, J. (1987). Declining serum concentrations of beta subunit of human chorionic gonadotropin and ruptured ectopic pregnancy. *American Journal of Obstetrics and Gynecology*, **156**: 940–943.

Gruft, L., Bertola, E., Luchini, L., Azzilonna, C., Bigatti, G., Parazzini, F (1994). Determinants of reproductive prognosis after ectopic pregnancy. *Human Reproduction*, **7**, 1333–1336.

Guirgis, R.R., Craft, I.L. (1991). Ectopic pregnancy resulting from gamete intrafallopian transfer and *in-vitro* fertilization. Role of ultrasonography in diagnosis and treatment. *Journal of Reproductive Medicine*, **36**(11): 793–796.

Johns, D.A., Hardy, R.P. (1986) Management of unruptured ectopic pregnancy with laparoscopic carbon dioxide laser. *Fertility and Sterility*, **46**: 703–705.

Johnson, N. (1993). Simplifying laparoscopic surgery for ectopic pregnancies. *British Journal of Obstetrics and Gynecology*, **100**: 286–287.

Koninckx, P.R., Witters, K., Brosens, J., Stemers, N., Oosterlynck, D., Meuleman, C. (1991). Conservative laparoscopic treatment of ectopic pregnancies using CO_2-laser. *British Journal of Obstetrics and Gynaecology*, **98**: 1254–1259.

Langer, R., Bukovsky, I., Herman, A., Ron–El., R., Lifshitz, Y., Caspi, E. (1987). Fertility following conservative surgery for tubal pregnancy. *Acta Obstetrica Gynecologica Scandinavica*, **66**(7): 649–652.

Levin, J.H., Lacarra, M., d'Ablaing, G., Grimes, D.A., Vermesh, M. (1990). Mifepristone (RU 486) failure in an ovarian heterotopic pregnancy. *American Journal of Obstetrics and Gynecology*, **163**(2): 543–544.

Loffer, F.D. (1986). Surgical settings and incisions for the management of ectopic pregnancy. *Journal of Reproductive Medicine*, **31**: 94–102.

Lund, J. (1955). Early ectopic pregnancy. Comments on conservative treatment. *Journal of Obstetrics and Gynaecology of the British Empire*, **62**: 70–76.

Lund, P.R., Sielaff, G.W., Aiman, E.J. (1989). *In-vitro* fertilization patient presenting in hemorrhagic shock caused by unsuspected heterotopic pregnancy. *American Journal of Emergency Medicine*, **7**(1): 49–53.

Lundorff, P., Hahlin, M., Sjoblom, P., Lindblom, B. (1991a). Persistent trophoblast after conservative treatment of tubal pregnancy: prediction and detection. *Obstetrics and Gynecology*, **77**: 129–133.

Lundorff, P., Thorburn, J., Hahlin, M., Kallfelt, B., Lindblom, B. (1991b). Adhesion formation after laparoscopic surgery in tubal pregnancy: a randomized trial versus laparotomy. *Fertility and Sterility*, **55**: 911–915.

McLain, P.L., Kirkwood, C.R. (1987). Ovarian and intrauterine heterotopic pregnancy following clomiphene ovulation induction: report of a healthy live birth. *Journal of Family Practice*, **24**(1): 76–79.

Magos, A.C., Baumann, R., Turnbull, A.C. (1988). Management of unruptured and ruptured ectopic pregnancies by videopelviscopy. *Lancet*, **2**: 275–276.

Magos, A.C., Baumann, R., Turnbull, A. C. (1989). Managing gynaecological emergencies with laparoscopy. *British Medical Journal*, **299**: 371–374.

Makinen, J.I., Kivijarvi, A.K., Irjala, K.M.A. (1990). Success of non-surgical management of ectopic pregnancy. *Lancet*, **1**: 1099.

Mashiach, S., Carp, H.J.A., Serr, D.M. (1982). Non-operative management of ectopic pregnancy. *Journal of Reproductive Medicine*, **27**: 27–32.

Mitchell, D. E., McSwain, H.F., Peterson, H.B. (1989). Fertility after ectopic pregnancy. *American Journal of Obstetrics and Gynecology*, **161**: 576–580.

Oelsner, G. (1987). Ectopic pregnancy in the sole remaining tube and the management of the patient with multiple ectopic pregnancies. *Clinical Obstetrics and Gynecology*, **30**(1): 225–229.

Oelsner, G., Rabinovitch, O., Morad, J., Mashiach, S., Serr, D.M. (1986). Reproductive outcome after microsurgical treatment of tubal pregnancy in women with a single fallopian tube. *Journal of Reproductive Medicine*, **31**: 483–486.

Ohel, G., Katz, M., Blumenthal, B. (1980). Complete abortion of early ectopic pregnancy. *International Journal of Gynecology and Obstetrics*, **17**: 596–597.

Pansky, M., Golan, A., Bukovsky, I., Caspi, E. (1991). Non-surgical management of tubal pregnancy. Necessity in view of the changing clinical appearance. *American Journal of Obstetrics and Gynecology*, **164**: 888–895.

Patton, G.W., Kistner, R.W. (1984). *Atlas of Infertility Surgery*, 2nd edn. Little Brown and Company, Boston.

Paulson, J.D., Asmar, P. (1989). Use of CO_2 laser surgery in the treatment of tubal pregnancy. In: *Ectopic Pregnancy: Pathophysiology and Clinical Management*, (eds C.M. Fredericks, J.D. Paulson, G. Holtz), pp. 141–151. Hemisphere, Washington.

Porter, R., Smith, B., Ahuja, K. (1986). Combined twin ectopic pregnancy and intrauterine gestation following *in-vitro* fertilization and embryo transfer. *Journal of in-vitro Fertilization and Embryo Transfer*, **3**: 330–332.

Pouly, J.L., Chapron, C., Canis, M., Mage, M., Wattiez, A., Manhes, H., Bruhat, M.A. (1991). Subsequent fertility for patients presenting with an ectopic pregnancy and having an intrauterine device *in situ*. *Human Reproduction*, **6**, 999–1001.

Pouly, J.L., Manhes, H., Mage, G. (1986). Conservative laparoscopic treatment of 321 ectopic pregnancies. *Fertility and Sterility*, **46**: 1093–1098.

Querleu, D., Boutteville, C. (1989). Fertility after ectopic pregnancy. *Fertility and Sterility*, **51** 1069–1070.

Rein, M.S., Di Salvo, D.N., Friedman, A.J. (1989). Heterotopic pregnancy associated with *in-vitro* fertilization and embryo transfer: a possible role for routine vaginal ultrasound. *Fertility and Sterility*, **51**(6): 1057–1058.

Sauer, M.V., Gorril, M.J., Rodi, I.A., Yeko, T.R., Greenberg, L.H., Bustillo, M., Gunning, J.E., Buster, J.E. (1987). Non-surgical management of unruptured ectopic pregnancy: an extended clinical trial. *Fertility and Sterility*, **48**: 752–755.

Saunders, N.J. (1990). Non-surgical treatment of ectopic pregnancy. *British Journal of Obstetrics and Gynaecology*, **97**: 972–973.

Semm, K. (1979). New methods of pelviscopy (gynecologic laparoscopy) for myomectomy, ovariectomy, tubectomy and adnectomy. *Endoscopy*, **11**: 85–89.

Sherman, D., Langer, R., Herman, A., Bukovsky, I., Caspi, E. (1987). Reproductive outcome after fimbrial evacuation of tubal pregnancy. *Fertility and Sterility*, **47**(3): 420–424.

Silva, P.D. (1988). A laparoscopic approach can be applied to most cases of ectopic pregnancy. *Obstetrics and Gynaecology*, **72**: 944–946.

Sondheimer, S.J., Tureck, R.W., Blasco, L. (1985). Simultaneous ectopic pregnancy with intrauterine twin gestations after *in-vitro* fertilization and embryo transfer. *Fertility and Sterility*, **43**: 313–319.

Stromme, W.B. (1973). Conservative surgery for ectopic pregnancy: a twenty years review. *Obstetrics and Gynecology*, **41**: 215–223.

Sultana, C.J., Easley, K., Collins, R.L., (1992). Outcome of laparoscopic versus traditional surgery for ectopic pregnancies. *Fertility and Sterility*, **57**: 285–289.

Taylor, P.J., Cumming, D.C. (1979). Combined laparoscopy and minilaparotomy in the management of unruptured tubal pregnancy: a preliminary report. *Fertility and Sterility*, **32**: 521–526.

Thorburn, J.E.K., Janson, P.O., Lindstedt, G. (1983). Early diagnosis of ectopic pregnancy. A review of 328 cases of a five year period. *Acta Obstetrica Gynecologica Scandinavica*, **62**: 543–549.

Thorburn, J.E.K., Philipson, M., Lindblom, B. (1988). Fertility after pregnancy in relation to background factors and surgical treatment. *Fertility and Sterility*, **49**, 595–601.

Thornton, K.L., Diamond, M.P., DeCherney, A.H. (1991). Linear salpingostomy for ectopic pregnancy. *Obstetrics and Gynecology Clinics of North America*, **18**: 95–110.

Timonen, S., Nieminen, U. (1967). Tubal pregnancy: choice of operative method of treatment. *Acta Obstetrica Gynecologica Scandinavica*, **46**: 327–329.

Tuomivaara, L., Kauppila, A. (1988). Radical or conservative surgery for ectopic pregnancy? A follow-up study of fertility of 323 patients. *Fertility and Sterility*, **50**, 580–583.

Valle, J.S., Lifchez, A.S. (1983). Reproductive outcome following conservative surgery for tubal pregnancy in women with a single fallopian tube. *Fertility and Sterility*, **39**: 316–320.

Vermesh, M., Presser, S.C. (1992). Reproductive outcome after linear salpingostomy for ectopic gestation: a prospective 3 year follow-up. *Fertility and Sterility*, **57**; 682–684.

Vermesh, M., Silva, P.D., Rosen, G.F., Stein, A.L., Fossum, G.T., Sauer, M.V. (1989). Management of unruptured ectopic gestation by linear salpingostomy: a prospective randomised clinical trial of laparoscopy versus laparotomy. *Obstetrics and Gynecology*, **73**: 400–403.

Winston, R.M.L., Margara, R.A. (1980). Techniques for the improvement of microsurgical tubal anastomosis. In: *Microsurgery in Female Infertility*. (eds: P.G. Grosignani, B.L. Rubin). Grune and Stratton, New York.

Yaffe, H., Navot, D., Laufer, N. (1979). Pitfalls in early detection of ectopic pregnancy. *Lancet*, 1: 227–229.

Ylostalo, P., Cacciatore, B., Sjoberg, J., Kaariainen, M., Tenhunen, A., Stenman, U. (1992). Expectant management of ectopic pregnancy. *Obstetrics and Gynecology*, **80**: 345–348.

Young, P.L., Saftlas, A.F., Atrash, H.K., Lawson, H.W., Petrey, F.F. (1991). National trends in the management of tubal pregnancy, 1970–1987. *Obstetrics and Gynecology*, **78**: 749–752.

Yovich, J.L., McColm, S.C., Turner, S.R., Matson, P.L. (1985). Heterotopic pregnancy from *in-vitro* fertilization. *Journal of in-vitro Fertilization and Embryo Transfer*, 2: 143–150.

Zacur, H.A. (1993). Expectant management of ectopic pregnancy. *Radiology*, **186**: 11–12.

Zouves, C., Urman, B., Gomel, V. (1992). Laparoscopic surgical treatment of tubal pregnancy. A safe effective alternative to laparotomy. *Journal of Reproductive Medicine*, **37**: 205–209.

CHAPTER 10

Radical Surgery

10.1 Introduction

The decision to treat ectopic pregnancy by means of a radical procedure should not be taken lightly. It is not a simple matter of ectopic pregnancy plus ruptured tube equals salpingectomy. Other factors, e.g. previous ectopic pregnancy, damaged or absent contralateral tube and future fertility requirements among others, should influence the surgical decision, which in any case needs to be discussed with the couple prior to surgery. The importance of these factors is exemplified by calculating the likelihood of an ectopic pregnancy re-occurring in a tube previously treated conservatively. In this case the incidence of ectopic pregnancy increases tenfold from approximately one in 100 to 200 in the general population to one in ten in women with a previous ectopic pregnancy or damaged tubes (Schoen and Nowak, 1975) and one in five future conceptions after two previous ectopic pregnancies (DeCherney *et al.*, 1985). It has been argued that unless the tube is irreparably damaged or bleeding is uncontrolled a conservative procedure should always be the first line treatment for ectopic pregnancy; only if this fails is a radical procedure required.

10.2 Choice of patients

There are few absolute indications for salpingectomy (Table 10.1). A desire for sterilisation is not generally accepted on its own as the primary indication for radical surgery, unless this has been documented in previous records. Relative indications are more difficult to list and the individual needs and desires of the couple should be considered. The most difficult decision is to judge whether the tube is severely or irreparably damaged. This can be assessed by estimating the length of the fallopian

Table 10.1. *Absolute and relative indications for salpingectomy*

Absolute indications	Relative indications
1. Treatment of EP which has irreparably damaged the tube	1. Severe but not irreparable damage to the tube
2. Control of bleeding	2. Repeat ectopic pregnancy in tube previously managed conservatively
(a) when patient is in shock	3. When fertility is no longer required
(b) during conservative management	4. To improve ovarian access in those planning or actively undergoing IVF-ET

EP, ectopic pregnancy; IVF-ET, *in-vitro* fertilisation-embryo transfer.

tube involved by the ectopic pregnancy, the health of the remaining non-involved tube (i.e. degree of scarring), extension into the mesosalpinx and damage to tubal blood vessels.

The management of a second pregnancy in the same tube previously treated conservatively is considered in Section 9.5.4. The repeat ectopic pregnancy rate is presumably much higher after two ectopics in the same tube than after only one. Most authors would therefore recommend a radical procedure (such as salpingectomy) in this situation, although the woman with no living children may opt for another conservative procedure, in the hope of a viable pregnancy.

10.3   Choice of operation

If a radical procedure is judged to be necessary (Table 10.1), three surgical options are available. The basic treatment is salpingectomy but this can be extended to include cornual resection and/or oophorectomy. Another option is bipolar tubal coagulation (or fulguration) in those patients with a small (less than 1.5 cm) ectopic pregnancy who wish to be sterilised. This can be performed by laparoscopy. The main disadvantage is that no specimen is available for histological confirmation of the diagnosis.

10.3.1   SALPINGECTOMY

In most cases salpingectomy is carried out at laparotomy, although enthusiasts have described successful outcomes after laparoscopic salpingectomy in patients with a small ectopic pregnancy (less than 2–3 cm in diameter), when bleeding is easily controlled, and when the pregnancy is not cornual. Experience with the technique is also an important determining factor (Semm, 1979). The procedure may require more than the standard two entry technique and the appropriate equipment must be available. The tube can be removed by laparoscopy using specially designed ligatures, such as those described by one of the pioneers of this technique, Kurt Semm. Once the blood supply to the tube is controlled by these ligatures, the tube is excised using a knife or scissors, again via the laparoscope. The tissue is then removed through the trochar channel of the laparoscope. Any remaining fragments are picked up individually using a morcellator. Others have suggested removing larger pieces of tissue via a colpotomy incision (Reich *et al.*, 1987). Alternatively diathermy or, if available, a laser could be used to cauterise the blood vessels to the tube and, if necessary, the ovary. The excised tissue is removed in the same way.

If a laparotomy is to be performed, the next decision is the type of incision. In most cases this will be a small (3–5 cm) Pfannensteil incision, although a vertical incision may be considered in the presence of a previous vertical incision and when there is a possibility that a different or an additional disease process (e.g. extensive adhesions) may require more extensive surgery.

When haemoperitoneum is associated with shock, rapid control of bleeding is required. In this situation, the uterus is grasped and brought up to the incision and the involved tube quickly identified. Haemostasis is effected by placing a clamp at the area of the utero-ovarian anastomosis and beneath and parallel to the involved tube. In the non-emergency situation, small clamps are placed across sections of the mesosalpinx progressing from the fimbrial to the cornual end of the tube. Each pedicle (which should not be excessively thick) is first incised using knife, scissors or diathermy, according to availability and surgical preference, and then tied off with fine resorbable suture material, e.g. 3.0 or 4.0 dexon. Once haemostasis is ensured, the abdomen is closed. Figure 10.1 depicts the appearance of the adnexae after bilateral salpingectomy.

10.3.2 OOPHORECTOMY

Ipsilateral oophorectomy may be indicated when the blood supply to the ovary is jeopardized, e.g., when rupture of the tube extends to the adjacent ovarian vessels. Every attempt should be made to preserve the ovary in case *in vitro* fertilisation-embryo transfer (IVF-ET) should

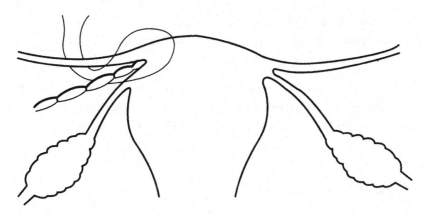

Figure 10.1 Appearance of the adnexae after bilateral salpingectomy.

subsequently be required for conception. The procedure is carried out in the standard manner by including the ovary in the pedicle of tissue to be removed with the tube. If the ovary is enlarged by a corpus luteum it may be necessary to take two or more bites of the pedicle with clamps to achieve haemostasis.

10.3.4 CORNUAL RESECTION

Some would advocate this procedure to reduce the length of a tube in which a future pregnancy can implant. It is performed by making an incision in the cornual region of the uterus using either a knife, cutting diathermy or laser and removing a cone or wedge of tissue with the tube at its base and the uterus at the apex. The next step is to oversew the cornual area and thus bury the lumen of the tube. As expected, the myometrial wall may be weakened by this procedure. It is therefore possible for the uterus to rupture in a subsequent pregnancy.

10.4 Point summary

1. Absolute indications for radical surgery include an irreparably damaged tube and bleeding control.

2. Treatment is salpingectomy (by laparoscopy or laparotomy) with or without cornual resection and/or oophorectomy.

3. The intrauterine pregnancy rate after radical surgery is approximately 45% with a 9% repeat ectopic pregnancy rate.

4. Irrespective of the surgical technique used, the condition of the contralateral tube and a history of infertilty are the most significant factors in terms of future fertility.

5. Women who have completed their families should be treated by salpingectomy rather than a conservative procedure because, although rare, the risk of complications is higher in the latter.

10.5   References

DeCherney, A.H., Sildker, J.S., Mezer, H.C.,Talatzis, B.C. (1985). Reproductive outcome following two ectopic pregnancies. *Fertility and Sterility,* **43**: 82–85.

Reich, H., Freifeld, M.L., McGlynn, F., Reich, E. (1987). Laparoscopic treatment of tubal pregnancy. *Obstetrics and Gynecology,* **69**: 275–279.

Schoen, J.A., Nowak, R.J. (1975). Repeat ectopic pregnancy. *Obstetrics and Gynecology,* **45**: 542–546.

Semm, K. (1979). New methods of pelviscopy (gynecologic laparoscopy) for myomectomy, ovariectomy, tubectomy and adnectomy. *Endoscopy,* **11**: 85–89.

CHAPTER 11

Pregnancy after ectopic pregnancy

11.1 Introduction

In this chapter we shall consider the outcome after treatment for ectopic pregnancy in terms of rates of conception, live births, abortions and recurrent ectopic pregnancy. One of the problems of reviewing reproductive performance after ectopic pregnancy is that there are numerous comparisons to be made, e.g. conservative versus radical surgery, laparoscopic versus open procedures at laparotomy, laser versus endoscopic techniques, salpingotomy versus segmental tubal resection or fimbrial expression. As elegantly described by Kadar (1990), many of the studies purporting to address this issue confuse these comparisons, such that meaningful conclusions cannot be easily drawn. In essence, what the practitioner needs to know is which procedure gives the best results in terms of future fertility, after allowance for other factors (quite apart from the surgical variables listed above) which are known to influence prognosis.

11.2 Precautions to be taken when analysing the results

Several precautions should be taken in analysing reproductive outcome data. These will be described by reference to the results of fimbrial evacuation (Langer et al., 1987; Sherman et al., 1987). First, two treatment modalities should be compared by intention to treat, rather than by actual treatment used. This principle is not always followed. For example, in the study by Sherman et al. (1987), 31 patients underwent successful fimbrial evacuation in a 13-year period; however, in an unspecified number the procedure was attempted but failed because of technical difficulties. These failed cases were treated by linear salpingotomy but were not included in the fimbrial evacuation series.

The second consideration is that of other abnormalities noted on examination of the pelvis. If adhesions and/or other tubal abnormalities are more common in one or other group, one would expect that group to have poorer subsequent outcome, irrespective of treatment modality. With notable exceptions (Sherman *et al.*, 1982; Thorburn *et al.*, 1988; Tuomivaara and Kauppila, 1988; Lundorff *et al.*, 1992; Ory *et al.*, 1993; Silva et al, 1993), this factor is not controlled for in the vast published database on subsequent pregnancy rates, summarised in Tables 11.1-11.3. This factor alone may explain the unusually low fertility rates, such as the 22% intrauterine pregnancy rate after laparoscopic salpingectomy reported by Dubuisson *et al.* (1990), which probably reflects distinctive patient characteristics such as a high proportion of patients with pre-existing infertility. Third, some patients may be excluded from follow-up for reasons which might include use of contraception, no intention to conceive or simply being lost to follow-up. This number should be clearly stated as well as the duration of follow-up. This point is illustrated by the series of Langer *et al.* (1987) and Sherman *et al.* (1987), in which potentially fertile patients treated by fimbrial expression were followed for a mean of 38 months (range 12–81 months). Twenty-five women conceived 39 times: 33 infants were liveborn (85%), with a 13% abortion rate. The authors are careful to state that this is the known abortion rate (spontaneous and induced); some women may have conceived and undergone an early complete abortion, of which they were not aware. There were no recurrent ectopic pregnancies in this series. Because of, or perhaps in spite of, these methodological limitations, these favourable data concerning fimbrial evacuation contrast sharply with the earlier data of Timonen and Niemenen (1967) that documented a much lower term pregnancy rate and repeat ectopic pregnancy rate (21%). High repeat ectopic pregnancy rates after fimbrial evacuation have also been reported by Swolin and Fall (1972), Bruhat *et al.* (1980), Paavonen *et al.* (1985) and Oelsner *et al.* (1987). It is noteworthy that, with a few exceptions, most of the recent papers report only intrauterine pregnancy rates, whereas most earlier studies (Ploman and Wicksell, 1960; Vehaskary *et al.*, 1960; Timonen and Nieminen, 1967; Swolin and Fall, 1972) documented the term or live birth rate, the figure which really interests our patients.

Table 11.1. *Reproductive outcome after conservative surgery*

Reference	No. of cases	IUP (%)[a]	REP (%)
Tompkins (1956)	6	50 (19)	33
Wexler et al. (1956)	79	29 (26)	4
Ploman and Wicksall (1960)	27	59 (NS)	18
Vehaskary (1960)	88	49 (30)	16
Grant (1962)	141	25 (19)	6
Stromme et al. (1962)	15	60 (NS)	0
Skulj et al. (1964)	92	NS (25)	1
Timonen and Nieminen (1967)	185	53 (24)	12
Jarvinen et al. (1972)	41	18 (14)	7
Swolin and Fall (1972)	24	12 (NS)	17
Stangel et al. (1977)	4	50 (50)	0
Janacek and DeGrandi (1978)	6	50 (50)	0
DeCherney and Kase (1979)	48	58 (39)	8
Buchovsky et al. (1979)	23	70 (NS)	1
Bruhat et al. (1980)	25	72 (NS)	12
Patton (1982)	17	53 (47)	11
Sherman et al. (1982)	104	72 (NS)	5
DeCherney et al. (1982)	15	73 (53)	20
Langer et al. (1982)	41	83 (73)	10
Sherman et al. (1982)	27	92 (85)	0
Paavonen et al. (1985)	39	51 (NS)	7
Corson and Batzer (1986)	96	35 (NS)	16
Oelsner et al. (1986)	22	66 (47)	42
Pouly et al. (1986)	118	64 (NS)	22
Cartwright et al. (1986)	8	38 (NS)	13
Hallatt (1986)	200	57 (NS)	14
Oelsner et al. (1987)	25	56 (NS)	12
Pouly et al. (1986)	118	64 (NS)	22
DeCherney and Diamond (1987)	69	52 (NS)	10
Reich et al. (1988)	38	50 (NS)	29
Silva (1988)	6	66 (NS)	0
Tulandi (1988)	24	50 (31)	19
Vermesh et al. (1989)	49	46 (NS)	11
Vermesh and Presser (1992)	60	57 (NS)	12
Silva et al. (1993)	52	54 (NS)	8

[a] Value in parenthesis is the term pregnancy rate
NS, not stated; IUP, intrauterine pregnancy; REP, repeat ectopic pregnancy.

Table 11.2. *Reproductive outcome following conservative surgery: a comparison of laparoscopy and abdominal salpingostomy*

Reference	Route	No. of cases	IUP (%)	REP (%)	Tubal patency on HSG (%)
Brumsted *et al.* (1988)	Laparoscopy	30	9/18 (50)	1/18 (6)	16/20 (80)
	Abdominal	30	8/19 (42)	3/19 (16)	17/19 (89)
Paulson and Asmar (1989)	Laparoscopy	22	6/16 (37)	5/16 (31)	19/19 (100)
	Abdominal	34	8/16 (50)	3/16 (18)	34/34 (100)
Koninckx *et al.* (1991)	Laparoscopy	34	17/34 (50)	NS	NS
	Abdominal	38	16/38 (42)	NS	NS
Vermesh and Presser (1992)	Laparoscopy	30	12/19 (63)	1/19 (5)	NS
	Abdominal	30	11/21 (52)	4/21 (19)	NS
Lundorff *et al.* (1992)	Laparoscopy	48	22/42 (52)	3/42 (7)	NS
	Abdominal	57	20/45 (44)	5/45 (11)	NS

NS, not stated; REP, repeat ectopic pregnancy; HSG, hysterosalpingography; IUP, intrauterine pregnancy.

11.3   Factors determining future prognosis

It is generally believed that fertility is lowered after surgery for ectopic pregnancy, although factors such as previous ectopic pregnancy, advanced age, and tubal adhesions are in themselves associated with reduced fertility rates and the increased risk of recurrent ectopic pregnancy (Kitchin *et al.*, 1984; Thorburn *et al.*, 1988; Pouly *et al.*, 1991b; Ory *et al.*, 1993). For example, in patients with a normal appearing contralateral tube, 80% reportedly have a subsequent viable pregnancy when treated by conservative surgery compared with a 55% viable pregnancy rate in those with periadnexal adhesions or a damaged contralateral tube (Langer *et al.*, 1982). Similarly, Sherman and colleagues (1982) reported that patients with a normal fertility history and normal pelvic findings had an 85% subsequent intrauterine pregnancy rate when managed by salpingotomy or salpingectomy. This compares favorably with the 44% intrauterine pregnancy rate in patients with an **abnormal** fertility history or abnormal findings at laparotomy treated by salpingectomy. By contrast, two larger and more recent studies (Tuomivaara and Kauppila, 1988; Gruft *et al.*, 1994) identified no significant asssociation between reproductive prognosis and age at surgery, parity, presence of adhesions in the contralateral tube or type of surgery.

It is logical that an unruptured tubal pregnancy would be less likely to hinder subsequent fertility than if the tube were to rupture. This appears to be borne out by the literature. In the study of Sherman and colleagues (1982), the subsequent intrauterine pregnancy rate was significantly higher (82%) in those whose ectopic pregnancy was managed prior to rupture compared with those who presented with a ruptured tube at surgery (65%). Similarly, if the pregnancy was viable or if the tubal gestation ends in complete abortion, the subsequent livebirth rate was higher (Timonen and Nieminen, 1967). Hence the impetus for early diagnosis and conservative treatment.

There is increasing evidence that of all these factors, a prior history of infertility may be the most significant determinant of fertility potential after laparotomy for ectopic pregnancy (Ory *et al.*, 1993). These authors observed that patients without prior infertility had a 68% term pregnancy rate, whether treated by conservative or radical surgery, compared with 25% and 11%, respectively, for those with a history of infertility. Although the study population of Ory *et al.* (1993) was quite small, they followed patients for at least three years or until conception occurred, thus providing realistic estimates of fertility potential. The results of this

Table 11.3. *Reproductive outcome after different procedures performed by the same route*

Reference	Procedure	No. of cases	IUP (%)	REP (%)
	Open			
Vehaskary (1960)	Salpingectomy	219	48	8
	Salpingostomy	88	49	16
Timonen and Nieminen (1967)	Salpingectomy	558	49	11
	Salpingostomy	185	53	12
DeCherney and Kase (1979)	Salpingectomy	50	42	12
	Salpingostomy	48	39	8
Swolin and Fall (1972)	Salpingectomy	44	12	16
	Salpingostomy	24	16	17
Ploman and Wicksell (1960)	Ablative	61	48	8
	Conservative	27	59	18
Sherman *et al.* (1982)	Ablative	104	72	5
	Conservative	47	83	6
	Closed			
Paavonen *et al.* (1985)	Salpingectomy	39	51	7
	Salpingostomy	34	53	9
Silva *et al.* (1993)	Salpingectomy	52	54	8
	Salpingostomy	80	60	18

IUP, intrauterine pregnancy; REP, repeat ectopic pregnancy.

study are consistent with the earlier findings of DeCherney and Kase (1979) that radical and conservative surgery offer comparable fertility potential and suggest that the choice of surgical procedure is not a significant determinant of fertility outcome in women with an ectopic pregnancy. As cautioned by the authors, these results should not be extrapolated to women managed by laparoscopic surgery.

Although not universally accepted, this observation supports the clinical recommendation described in Chapter 9, that conservative surgery, i.e. linear salpingotomy (tube closed) or salpingostomy (tube left open), is the treatment of choice in women desiring subsequent pregnancy. Women with a prior history of infertility have a poor subsequent fertility prognosis regardless of the procedure chosen. They should be advised to consider *in-vitro* fertilisation (IVF) (Ory *et al.*, 1993).

11.4   Fertility after ectopic pregnancy

11.4.1   OVERALL RESULTS

Fertility outcome after various treatment options is summarised in Tables 11.1 to 11.3. The end-points are recurrent ectopic pregnancy and subsequent intrauterine pregnancy rates. The therapeutic choice in any individual case depends, in part, on the balance of these two figures (Franklin *et al.*, 1973). This can be expressed in the form of the ectopic to intrauterine pregnancy ratio, which reflects the effectiveness of the treatment (Lundorff *et al.*, 1992).

One of the better studies in this field is that of Gruft *et al.* (1994) who examined the medical records of 265 women who underwent laparotomy for ectopic pregnancy between 1985 and 1990. These women had a 54% probability of subsequent pregnancy. This is broadly consistent with figures reported from several other countries (Toumivaara and Kauppila, 1988; Mitchell *et al.*, 1989; Querleu and Boutteville, 1989; Pouly *et al.*, 1991b) although the study of Sultana *et al.* (1992) reported a pregnancy rate of approximately 20%, presumably because their study included all patients and not only those who wished to become pregnant. Gruft *et al.* (1994) reported a 36% likelihood of giving birth to a child (cumulative live birth rate) during the three years after surgery, this value falling to 7% after one previous ectopic pregnancy. This is consistent with the work from other centres which demonstrate that the number of previous ectopic pregnancies is one of the major determinants of reproductive prognosis (Thorburn *et al.*, 1988; Querleu and Boutteville, 1989).

11.4.2   CONSERVATIVE TREATMENT

The philosophy behind conservative treatment is that preserving the tube increases the chance of subsequent live births (Valle and Lifchez, 1983). Recent studies have shown that fertility after conservative treatment of an ectopic pregnancy by salpingostomy is similar whether carried out via laparoscopy or laparotomy (Table 11.2). The results of conservative surgery suggest that, irrespective of the surgical technique used, the condition of the contralateral tube and a history of infertility are the most significant factors in determining future fertility. Unfortunately, comparison between the numerous published series is hampered by the fact that some have grouped together patients in whom the contralateral tube was normal and abnormal, and most do not specify whether their patients were previously infertile or not.

Moreover, since a subsequent pregnancy may occur through either the presumed normal tube or through the one previously operated, it is difficult to evaluate whether the conservative procedure was indeed successful. Perhaps the best way to do this is to examine pregnancy rates in women who have a single tube present (Jarvinen *et al.*, 1972; Stromme, 1973; Langer *et al.*, 1982; DeCherney *et al.*, 1982; Valle and Lifchez, 1983; Hallatt, 1986; Pouly *et al.*, 1986; Oelsner *et al.*, 1987; Tulandi, 1988). Term pregnancy rates in women wishing to become pregnant range from 20% in five women (Stromme, 1973) to 100% in 11 women (Valle and Lifchez, 1983). The reader should note that fewer than 35 term pregnancies have been reported in these series. The repeat ectopic pregnancy rate ranged from 0% (Valle and Lifchez, 1983) to 40% (Stromme, 1973). Oelsner et al (1986) pointed out that the worst outcome appears to be in those women treated conservatively after a previous tuboplasty. Three of the five women with a single tube treated conservatively had a repeat ectopic pregnancy, one spontaneously aborted in the first trimester and the last failed to conceive. They suggest that conservative procedures should be avoided in such women. Although these numbers are very small, most gynaecologists would consider treating ectopic pregnancy located in the woman's only remaining tube by salpingostomy, although the advent of assisted reproductive techniques may offer these women another option (Sections 9.5.4 and 11.5). Few today would remove or ligate diseased tubes prophylactically in an attempt to prevent ectopic pregnancies (Tucker *et al.*, 1981; Hewitt *et al.*, 1985), perhaps because pregnancies do occur in spontaneous cycles after IVF. Moreover, this procedure cannot prevent cornual or interstitial pregnancy.

Although the reproductive outcome after conservative surgery is reasonably well defined (approximately 50% subsequent pregnancies and 15% recurrent ectopic pregnancies), the situation becomes less clear when specific treatment options are compared (Tuomivaara and Kauppila, 1988; Mecke *et al.*, 1989; Pouly *et al.*, 1991a; Sultana *et al.*, 1992; Gruft *et al.*, 1994). This is described in the sections that follow.

11 4.3 CONSERVATIVE SURGERY: LAPAROSCOPY VERSUS LAPAROTOMY

Several retrospective case controlled studies have addressed the issue of reproductive outcome after a conservative procedure performed by laparoscopy or at open surgery (Table 11.2). More recently, a prospective randomised study comparing fertility outcome after salpingotomy at laparotomy versus laparoscopy has been reported (Lundorff *et al.*, 1992). Amongst 87 women desirous of pregnancy after conservative treatment of an ectopic pregnancy, there was no difference in the overall fertility outcome between the two groups (59% and 55%, respectively). Intrauterine pregnancy rates were significantly lower in the subgroup without bilateral tubal patency (26%) compared with those in whom contralateral patency had been demonstrated (60%). Thus, contrary to the findings of Bruhat *et al.* (1980), laparoscopic salpingotomy did not appear to improve future fertility in this study. A note of caution should be sounded in interpreting these results: patients in both groups were operated upon by surgeons trained in tuboplasty and microsurgery using atraumatic techniques. The results may not be equally applicable to a group of patients managed by gynaecologists of varying expertise. Moreover, quite apart from reproductive outcome, there is now convincing evidence that there are economic and cosmetic advantages to laparoscopic procedures (Brumsted *et al.*, 1988; Magos *et al.*, 1989; Vermesh *et al.*, 1989).

11.4.4 CONSERVATIVE VERSUS RADICAL TREATMENT

Reproductive outcome after all forms of conservative surgery reported over the last few decades is summarised in Table 11.1. Documented subsequent intrauterine pregnancy rates in these 35 studies on several hundred conservative operations of varying types (salpingostomy, salpingotomy, fimbrial evacuation or mid-tubal resection), range from 12% to 92%; repeat ectopic pregnancies occurred in 0 to 42% of patients. Although the studies are not uniform, approximately 50% of patients will have a subsequent intrauterine pregnancy and 12% a repeat ectopic pregnancy after conservative surgery.

Table 11.3 summarises the reproductive outcome of conservative versus radical treatment of ectopic pregnancy as published in the literature. Reported subsequent intrauterine pregnancy rates after radical surgery vary from 12% to 72% and the incidence of repeat ectopic pregnancy ranges from 5% to 16%. These wide variations arise from the differences in reporting characteristics described in Section 11.2. By calculating the incidence of pregnancy as a percentage of all patients who were operated on, it is possible to underestimate the true incidence; however, by using the number of women who desire pregnancy after a radical procedure as the denominator, approximately 45% of women will have a subsequent term pregnancy and 9% will have a repeat ectopic pregnancy (Lavy *et al.*, 1987).

As clearly illustrated in Table 11.3, the live birth rate after radical procedures is not significantly different from that after conservative surgery, whereas the repeat ectopic pregnancy rate is higher after conservative procedures; however, because of the small numbers of patients involved, these data do not reach statistical significance. When studies control for some of the major determinants of reproductive outcome, such as disease in the contralateral tube, the intrauterine pregnancy rate appears to be higher after conservative than radical procedures (Sherman *et al.*, 1982; Tuomivaara and Kauppila, 1988). Thorburn *et al.* (1988) have clearly shown that patient characteristics are of greater importance than the operative treatment chosen in determining subsequent reproductive outcome.

When both tubes are present, ectopic pregnancy is as likely to re-occur in the opposite, presumably normal, tube as in the tube operated on conservatively (DeCherney and Kase, 1979; DeCherney *et al.*, 1985; Hallatt, 1986; Pouly *et al.*, 1986; DeCherney and Diamond, 1987; Reich *et al.*, 1988). The rate of recurrent ectopic pregnancy in relation to the presence or absence of disease in the contralateral tube has not been examined. The World collaborative report on IVF pregnancies reported that recurring ectopic pregnancies accounted for 1.7% of pregnancies and 0.23% of embryo transfers (Cohen *et al.*, 1986).

11.5   What do these results mean?

Bearing in mind the limitations of treatment comparisons, a number of questions remain unanswered. One of the most important is whether the gynaecologist should perform a conservative procedure or not. The available evidence suggests that every attempt should be made to save the tube if the woman wishes future fertility and either the contralateral tube appears diseased (or is known to be blocked) or she has only one remaining tube. The reason that a conservative procedure is deemed inadvisable when the contralateral tube is normal, is that the live birth rate after radical procedures is not significantly different from that after conservative surgery, whereas the repeat ectopic pregnancy rate is higher after conservative procedures. By removing the affected tube, however, the treatment options available to that patient have been reduced should the ectopic pregnancy recur. Most clinicians are guided in their decision to conserve the unruptured tube or not by the size of the gestation. In practice, most would attempt salpingostomy whenever a small ectopic pregnancy is located in an unruptured tube regardless of whether the contralateral adnexa is normal or abnormal. Should complications occur during salpingostomy, the patient with a normal contralateral adnexa is more likely to be treated by salpingectomy than the patient with contralateral tubal disease.

11.6   Point summary

1. After conservative surgery, approximately 50% of patients will have a subsequent intrauterine pregnancy, 40% a live birth and 12% a repeat ectopic pregnancy.

2. Fertility rates after salpingotomy via laparoscopy or laparotomy are similar.

3. The intrauterine pregnancy rate after radical procedures (45%) is not significantly different to that after conservative surgery, but the repeat ectopic pregnancy rate is lower (9%).

4. Recurrent ectopic pregnancy is as likely to occur in the opposite, presumably normal tube, as in the tube operated on conservatively.

5. Women who undergo salpingostomy or salpingotomy for an ectopic pregnancy located in their only fallopian tube have a live birth rate of approximately 40% and a repeat ectopic pregnancy rate of 20%.

6. The presence of risk factors such as prior tubal disease, previous ectopic pregnancy or a history of infertility reduces the likelihood of intrauterine pregnancy and increases the chance of recurrent ectopic pregnancy.

11.7   References

Bruhat, M.A., Manhes, H., Mage, G., Pouly, J.L. (1980). Treatment of ectopic pregnancy by means of laparoscopy. *Fertility and Sterility*, **33**: 411–414.

Brumsted, J., Kessler, C., Gibson, C., Nakajima, S., Riddick, D.H., Gibson, M. (1988). A comparison of laparoscopy and laparotomy for the treatment of ectopic pregnancy. *Obstetrics and Gynaecology*, **71**: 889–892.

Buchovsky, I., Langer, R., Herman, A. (1979). Conservative surgery for tubal pregnancy. *Obstetrics and Gynecology*, **53**: 709–712.

Cartwright, P., Herbert, C.M., Maxson, W.S. (1986). Operative laparoscopy for the management of tubal pregnancy. *Journal of Reproductive Medicine,* **31**: 589–591.

Cohen, J., Mayaux, M.J., Guihard-Moscato, M.L., Schwartz, D. (1986). *In vitro* fertilization and embryo transfer: A collaborative study of 1163 pregnancies on the incidence and risk factors of ectopic pregnancies. *Human Reproduction,* **1**: 255–258.

Corson, S.L., Batzer, F.R. (1986). Ectopic pregnancy: a review of the etiologic factors. *Journal of Reproductive Medicine,* **31**: 78–85.

DeCherney, A.H., Diamond, M.P. (1987). Laparoscopic salpingostomy for ectopic pregnancy. *Obstetrics and Gynaecology,* **70**: 948–950.

DeCherney, A.H., Kase, N. (1979). The conservative surgical management of unruptured ectopic pregnancy. *Obstetrics and Gynaecology,* **54**: 451–454.

DeCherney, A.H., Maheaux, R., Naftolin, F. (1982). Salpingostomy for ectopic pregnancy in the sole patent oviduct: Reproductive outcome. *Fertility and Sterility,* **37**: 619–622.

DeCherney, A.H., Silidkes, J.S., Mezes, H.C., Tarlatzis, B.C. (1985). Reproductive outcome following two ectopic pregnancies. *Fertility and Sterility,* **43**: 82–89.

Dubuisson, J.B., Aubriot, F.X., Foulot, H., Bruel, D., Bouquet de Joliniere, J., Mandelbrot, L. (1990). Reproductive outcome after laparoscopic salpingectomy for tubal pregnancy. *Fertility and Sterility,* **53**: 1004–1007.

Franklin, E.W., Zeiderman, A.M., Lammele, P. (1973). Tubal ectopic pregnancy: etiology, obstetric and gynaecologic sequelae. *American Journal of Obstetrics and Gynaecology,* **117**: 220–225.

Grant, A. (1962). The effect of ectopic pregnancy on fertility. *Clinical Obstetrics and Gynecology,* **5**: 853–855.

Gruft, L., Bertola, E., Luchini, L., Azzilonna, C., Bigatti, G., Parazzini, F. (1994). Determinants of reproductive prognosis after ectopic pregnancy. *Human Reproduction,* **7**: 1333–1336.

Hallatt, J.G. (1986). Tubal conservatism in ectopic pregnancy: a study of 200 cases. *American Journal of Obstetrics and Gynaecology,* **154**: 1216–1221.

Hewitt, J., Martin, R., Steptoe, P.C., Rowland, U.F., Webster, J. (1985). Bilateral tubal ectopic pregnancy following in vitro fertilization and embryo replacement. *British Journal of Obstetrics and Gynaecology,* **92**: 850–852.

Janacek, P., DeGrandi, P. (1978). Chirurgie restauratrice d'emblee dand le traitment des grossesses extrauterines. *Journal Gynecology Obstetrics Reproductive Biology,* **7**: 1261–1265.

Jarvinen, P.A., Nummi, S., Pietila, K. (1972). Conservative operative treatment of tubal pregnancy with postoperative daily hydrotubations.

Acta Obstetrica Gynecologica Scandinava, **51**: 169–170.

Kadar, N. (1990). *Diagnosis and Treatment of Extrauterine pregnancies*. Raven Press: New York.

Kitchin, J.D., Wein, R.M, Nunley, W.C. Jr., Thiagarajah, S., Thornton, W.N. (1984). Ectopic pregnancy: current clinical trends. *American Journal of Obstetrics and Gynaecology*, **134**: 870–874.

Koninckx, P.R., Witters, K., Brosens, J., Stemers, N., Oosterlynck, D., Meuleman, C. (1991). Conservative laparoscopic treatment of ectopic pregnancies using CO_2-laser. *British Journal of Obstetrics and Gynecology*, **98**: 1254–1259.

Langer, R., Bukovsky, I., Herman, A., Ron-El, R., Lifshitz, Y., Caspi, E. (1987). Fertility following conservative surgery for tubal pregnancy. *Acta Obstetrica Gynecologica Scandinava*, 66(7): 649–652.

Langer, R., Bukovsky, I., Herman, A., Sherman, D., Sadovski, G., Caspi, E. (1982). Conservative surgery for tubal pregnancy. *Fertility and Sterility*, **38**: 427–430.

Lavy, G., Diamond, M.P., DeCherney, A.H. (1987). Ectopic pregnancy: its relationship to tubal reconstructive surgery. *Fertility and Sterility*, **47**: 543–546.

Lundorff, P., Thorburn, J., Lindblom, B. (1992). Fertility outcome after conservative surgery treatment of ectopic pregnancy evaluated in a randomized trial. *Fertility and Sterility*, **57**: 998–1002.

Magos, A.C., Baumann, R., Turnbull, A. C. (1989). Managing gynaecological emergencies with laparoscopy. *British Medical Journal*, **299**: 371–374.

Mecke, H., Semm, K., Lehmann-Willenbrock, E. (1989). Results of operative pelviscopy in 202 cases of ectopic pregnancy. *International Journal of Fertility*, **34**: 93–100.

Mitchell, D.E., McSwain, H.F., Peterson, H.B. (1989). Fertility after ectopic pregnancy. *American Journal of Obstetrics and Gynecology*, **161**: 576–580.

Oelsner, G. (1987). Ectopic pregnancy in the sole remaining tube and the management of the patient with multiple ectopic pregnancies. *Clinical Obstetrics and Gynecology*, **30**(1): 225–229.

Oelsner, G., Morad, J., Carp, H., Serr, D.M. (1987). Reproductive performance following conservative microsurgical management of tubal pregnancy. *British Journal of Obstetrics and Gynaecology*, **94**: 1078–1083.

Oelsner, G., Rabinovitch, O., Morad, J., Mashiach, S., Serr, D.M. (1986). Reproductive outcome after microsurgical treatment of tubal pregnancy in women with a single fallopian tube. *Journal of Reproductive Medicine*, **31**: 483–486.

Ory, S.J., Nnadi, E., Herrmann, R., O'Brien, P.S., Melton, L.J. (1993). Fertility after ectopic pregnancy. *Fertility and Sterility*, **60**: 231–235.

Paavonen, J., Varjonen-Toivonen, M., Komulainen, M., Heinonen, P.K. (1985). Diagnosis and management of tubal pregnancy: effect on fertility outcome. *International Journal of Gynecology and Obstetrics*, **23**: 129–133.

Patton, G.W. (1982) Pregnancy outcome following microsurgical fimbrioplasty. *Fertility and Sterility*, **37**: 150–155.

Paulson, J.D., Asmar, P. (1989). Use of CO_2 laser surgery in the treatment of tubal pregnancy. In: *Ectopic Pregnancy: Pathophysiology and Clinical Management*, eds C.M. Fredericks, J.D. Paulson, and G. Holtz. pp. 141–151. Hemisphere: Washington.

Ploman, L., Wicksell, F. (1960). Fertility after conservative surgery in tubal pregnancy. *Acta Obstetrica Gynaecologica Scandinava*, **39**: 143–152.

Pouly, J.L., Manhes, H., Mage, G. (1986). Conservative laparoscopic treatment of 321 ectopic pregnancies. *Fertility and Sterility*, **46**: 1093–1097.

Pouly, J.L., Chapron, C., Canis, M., Mage, M., Wattiez, A., Manhes, H., Bruhat, M.A. (1991a). Subsequent fertility for patients presenting with an ectopic pregnancy and having an intrauterine device *in situ*. *Human Reproduction*, **6**: 999–1001.

Pouly, J.L., Chapron, C., Manhes, H., Canis, M., Wattiez, A. (1991b). Multifactorial analysis of fertility after conservative laparoscopic treatment of ectopic pregnancy in a series of 223 patients. *Fertility and Sterility*, **56**: 453–460.

Querleu, D., Boutteville, C. (1989). Fertility after ectopic pregnancy. *Fertility and Sterility*, **51**: 1069–1070.

Reich, H., Johns, D.A., DeCaprio, J., McGlynn, F., Reich, E. (1988). Laparoscopic treatment of 109 consecutive ectopic pregnancies. *Journal of Reproductive Medicine*, **33**: 885–887.

Sherman, D., Langer, R., Herman, A., Bukovsky, I., Caspi, E. (1987). Reproductive outcome after fimbrial evacuation of tubal pregnancy. *Fertility and Sterility*, **47**(3): 420–424.

Sherman, D., Langer, R., Sadovsky, G., Bukovsky, I., Caspi, E. (1982). Improved fertility following ectopic pregnancy. *Fertility and Sterility*, **37**: 497–502.

Silva, P.D. (1988). A laparoscopic approach can be applied to most cases of ectopic pregnancy. *Obstetrics and Gynecology*, **72**: 944–946.

Silva, P.A., Schaper, A.M., Rooney, B. (1993). Reproductive outcome after 143 laparoscopic procedures for ectopic pregnancy. *Obstetrics and Gynecology*, **81**: 710–715.

Skulj, V., Pavlic, Z., Stoiljkovic, C. (1964). Conservative operative treatment of tubal pregnancy. *Fertility and Sterility*, **15**: 634–636.

Stangel, J.J., Reyniak, J.V., Stone, M.L. (1977). Conservative surgical management of tubal pregnancy with tubal reconstruction. *Surgical Forum*, **28**: 577–578.

Stromme, W.B. (1973). Conservative surgery for ectopic pregnancy: a twenty years review. *Obstetrics and Gynecology,* **41**: 215–223.

Stromme, W.B., McKelvey, J.L, Adkins, C.D. (1962). Conservative surgery for ectopic pregnancy. *Obstetrics and Gynecology,* **19**: 294–296.

Sultana, C.J., Easley, K., Collins, R.L. (1992). Outcome of laparoscopic versus traditional surgery for ectopic pregnancies. *Fertility and Sterility,* **57**: 285–289.

Swolin, K., Fall, M. (1972). Ectopic pregnancy. *Acta European Fertility,* **3**: 147–157.

Thorburn, J., Philipson, M., Lindblom, B. (1988). Fertility after pregnancy in relation to background factors and surgical treatment. *Fertility and Sterility,* **49**: 595–601.

Timonen, S., Nieminen, U. (1967). Tubal pregnancy: choice of operative method of treatment. *Acta Obstetrica Gynecologica Scandinavica,* **46**: 327–329.

Tompkins, P. (1956). Preservation of fertility by conservative surgery for ectopic pregnancy. *Fertility and Sterility,* **7**: 448–451.

Tucker, M., Smith, D.H., Pike, I., Kemp, J.F., Picker, R.H., Saunde, D.M. (1981). Ectopic pregnancy following in vitro fertilization and embryo transfer. *Lancet,* **1**: 1278.

Tulandi, T. (1988). Reproductive performance of women after two tubal ectopic pregnancies. *Fertility and Sterility,* **50**: 164–166.

Tuomivaara, L., Kauppila, A. (1988). Radical or conservative surgery for ectopic pregnancy? A follow-up study of fertility of 323 patients. *Fertility and Sterility,* **50**: 580–583.

Valle, J.S., Lifchez, A.S. (1983). Reproductive outcome following conservative surgery for tubal pregnancy in women with a single fallopian tube. *Fertility and Sterility,* **39**: 316–320.

Vehaskary, A. (1960). The operation of choice for ectopic pregnancy with reference to subsequent fertility. *Acta Obstetrica Gynecologica Scandinavica,* **39**(Suppl. 13): 3–11.

Vermesh, M., Presser, S.C. (1992). Reproductive outcome after linear salpingostomy for ectopic gestation: a prospective 3 year follow-up. *Fertility and Sterility,* **57**: 682–684.

Vermesh, M., Silva, P.D., Rosen, G.F., Stein, A.L., Fossum, G.T., Sauer, M.V. (1989). Management of unruptured ectopic gestation by linear salpingostomy: a prospective randomised clinical trial of laparoscopy versus laparotomy. *Obstetrics and Gynecology,* **73**: 400–403.

Wexler, D.J., Kohn, A., Birnberg, C.H. (1956). Conservative tubal surgery in ectopic pregnancy. *Fertility and Sterility,* **7**: 241–245.

The future

If one were to speculate as to which aspects of the diagnosis and management of ectopic pregnancy are most likely to undergo radical change in the next decade, one could reasonably suggest two main areas:

1. Advances in fibreoptics allowing for ever more ingenious and adventurous attempts to cannulate the fallopian tube with a view to non-traumatic diagnosis and gentle treatment.

2. The possibility of successfully re-locating ectopic pregnancy to the uterine cavity. This has been attempted several times in the last century, the earliest recorded attempt being ascribed to Wallace in 1917 who described a successful case following coincidental detection of ectopic pregnancy in a woman undergoing laparotomy for uterine fibroids. More recently, Shettles (1990) described successful re-implantation of a 40-day-old gestational sac using a glass tube pushed through the myometrium until decidua was obtained by gentle suction. A third published case via the cervical route has been contested (Pearce et al., 1994). Numerous other attempts using the transcervical technique have failed (F. Forsdahl, J.G. Westergaard, J.G. Grudzinskas, personal communication). Grudzinskas et al. (1994) have suggested that provided certain prerequisites are fulfilled, such as facilities for accurate and early diagnosis of ectopic pregnancy, counselling for potential recruits, on-call surgical and embryology teams, availability of rapid and accurate karyotyping techniques, and progress in the development of suitable surgical technique for the removal and re-location of the pregnancy, this may be a worthwhile technique to explore.

References

Grudzinskas, J.G., Palomino, M., Amstrong, P., Lowes, A. (1994). Relocation of ectopic pregnancy to the uterine cavity: a dream or reality? *British Journal of Obstetrics and Gynaecology*, **101**, 651–653.

Pearce, M., Manyonda, I.T., Chamberlain, G.V.P. (1994). Term delivery after intrauterine relocation of an ectopic pregnancy. *British Journal of Obstetrics and Gynaecology*, **101**: 716–717.

Shettles, L.B. (1990). Tubal embryo successfully transferred *in utero*. *American Journal of Obstetrics and Gynecology*, **163**: 2026–2027.

Wallace, C.J. (1917). Transplantation of ectopic pregnancy from fallopian tube in cavity of uterus. *Surgery, Gynecology and Obstetrics*, **24**: 578–579.

INDEX

Entries in *italics* refer to illustrations. In some cases there are textual references on these pages.

Printed in the United States
By Bookmasters